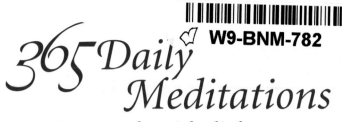

365 Daily Meditations
For people with diabetes

Catherine Feste

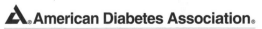

American Diabetes Association.
Cure • Care • Commitment®

Director, Book Publishing, John Fedor; Associate Director, Consumer Books, Sherrye Landrum; Editor, Sherrye Landrum; Associate Director, Book Production, Peggy M. Rote; Composition, Circle Graphics, Inc.; Cover Design, Koncept Inc.; Printer, Versa Press, Inc.

Printed in the United States of America
1 3 5 7 9 10 8 6 4 2

⊗ The paper in this publication meets the requirements of the ANSI Standard Z39.48-1992 (permanence of paper).

ADA titles may be purchased for business or promotional use or for special sales. To purchase this book in large quantities, or for custom editions of this book with your logo, contact Lee Romano Sequeira, Special Sales & Promotions, at the address below, or at LRomano@diabetes.org or 703-299-2046.

American Diabetes Association
1701 North Beauregard Street
Alexandria, Virginia 22311

Library of Congress Cataloging-in-Publication Data
Feste, Catherine.
    365 daily meditations for people with diabetes / Catherine Feste.
       p. cm.
    ISBN 1-58040-145-7 (pbk.)
    1. Diabetes—Popular works. 2. Diabetes—Psychological aspects. 3.
Diabetes—Quotations, maxims, etc. I. Title: Three hundred sixty-five meditations for
People with diabetes. II. Title.

RC660.4.F468 2004
616.4'62—dc22   2004050919

Dedication

For her wisdom, faith, and never-ending support, this book is lovingly dedicated to my mother

C. Eleanor Nelson
1916–2003

Contents

Foreword

It is only quite recently that illness has been defined as a function of the body. At the beginnings of medicine, the shamans or medicine men defined illness not in terms of pathology but in terms of the soul. In this older wisdom, illness is "soul loss," a loss of direction, purpose, meaning, mystery, and awe. According to these ancients, the healing from illness required an attention to the realm of spirit, a recovery of the soul.

What then is spirit? Spirit is the basis for the value of every human life, the source of our dignity, and the foundation of our experience of integrity, despite bodily changes. The capacity for spiritual experience is so universal that every language has its own name for it: the Atman, the Neshuma, the Ra, the Ru-ach, the Divine Spark. We call this capacity the soul.

Illness and suffering draw the soul and its issues closer. Everything I have learned about spirit I have learned from listening to people with cancer in my work as a physician and from my long and personal experience with Crohn's disease, a chronic illness of the intestine.

These experiences have taught me that spirit is not just a human capacity, it is a human need. This seems especially true in times of loss, in times of illness and crisis. At such times, spirit is strength.

The pursuit of meaning is often the doorway to the spirit. The language of the soul is meaning. In the setting of a chronic illness, people instinctively reach for personal meaning, people who have never considered this dimension of life before. Meaning helps us to see in the dark. It strengthens the will to live in us.

Our sense of the meaning of a common event is as unique as our fingerprints: an illness like diabetes will mean something different to every person who is touched by it. Many years ago when I went to medical school, the meaning of an illness was seen as irrelevant. But we did not know much about healing then. Our focus was on cure. While cure happens to the body, healing happens to the whole person. Many things that are beyond cure can still heal. I suppose one might even say that there is a healthy way to have a disease, a way to use this difficult experience to come to know intimately the value and meaning of your life.

Experiencing spirit and meaning does not require us to live differently. Many of us already live far more meaningful lives than we realize. Experiencing meaning often requires a shift in perspective, the development of new eyes. Finding meaning is about seeing beyond the superficial and the obvious to the essential. Seeing the ordinary and the familiar in new ways. Meaning does not change the events of our lives, it changes our experience of those events. It may be the difference between seeing yourself as a victim and seeing yourself as a hero.

Through illness, people may come to know themselves for the first time, to recognize not only who they really are but what really matters. Illness shuffles the hierarchy of our values like a deck of cards. Often a value that has been on the bottom of the deck for years turns out to be the top card. In illness, people abandon values they inherited with their family name, values that they have never questioned before, and uncover ways of living far more genuine and unique. Often these ways are also more soul-infused. In all the years that I have listened to people with cancer, no one has ever said to me that if they died, they would miss their Mercedes, even though such a car and all that it represents has been the focus of their lives for many years. This shift may represent a kind of healing.

Illness often naturally initiates a movement toward greater wholeness. In the 25 years that I have been a physician to people with cancer, I have witnessed this many times over. I have been with people as they have discovered in themselves an unexpected strength, a courage beyond what they would have thought possible, an unsuspected sense of compassion, and a capacity for love far deeper than they had ever dreamed.

When I first became ill with my own chronic illness more than 45 years ago, I felt profoundly diminished, different, and even ashamed. I had not known then that what challenges the body can evolve and strengthen the soul. I had focused on the curing of my body. It took years for me to recognize the movement toward wholeness that had happened in me while my attention was elsewhere—to know that it is possible to live a good life even if it is not an easy life.

Curing is about the recovery of the body. Healing is about the recovery of the soul. Science cures us. Meaning heals us. Some years ago I wrote this poem about my own experience of illness:

O
Body!
For 45 years,
1,573 experts with a combined
14,355 years of training

have failed
to
cure
your
wounds.

Deep inside,
I
am
whole.

The capacity for spirit and meaning are a part of
our birthright as human beings. My experience as
both physician and patient has led me to believe that
illness is often an awakening and a spiritual path.
There are many ways to travel this path, to move
toward our wholeness, and strengthen the innate
spirit in us. Meditations on Diabetes offers us a wide
variety of such approaches, and I am honored to be
asked to introduce this book to you. It is a book of wisdom for the path, and a gift to those whose lives have
been touched by diabetes. It will help anyone who
reads it to use the experience of illness to deepen and
enrich the experience of life.

Rachel Naomi Remen, MD
Author, *Kitchen Table Wisdom: Stories that Heal*
and *My Grandfather's Blessings.*

Acknowledgments

From the beginning, this project has been surrounded by love and guided by a wide and wonderful variety of angels. Their contributions included serving as a sounding board as I tried out the thoughts that became foundational to the book. Some of them served as reviewers and shared helpful comments and insights. Several of the messages I used came from messenger angels listed here. I acknowledge these people and their contributions to this book and to my life: Mark Anderson, Anne Carlson, Mary Casey, Sheila Folkestad, Lyle Gerard, Dick and Diana Guthrie, Mary Jackson, Delores Kanten, Judy Louden, Terry Morehouse, Jan Norman, Jan Olson, Ginny Peragallo-Dittko, Kathy Plumb, Ellen Reeder, Dawn Satterfield, Rich and Linda Sedgwick, Dan Schindler, Jen Smith, Ruth Stricker, and Nancy Youngdahl.

Special thanks to Sherrye Landrum, my wonderful editor, whose enthusiasm, encouragement, and guidance were critical to the writing of this book.

And, a special word of thanks to my long-time friend and mentor, Bob Esbjornson. He shared his important perspectives as religion professor, medical ethicist, husband, and father of people who have diabetes, and he shared his beautiful soul. Thanks, Esbj.

For their remarkable and inspiring leadership in the field of healing and spirituality, I owe a heartfelt and profound "thank you" to Dr. MaryJo Kreitzer, Director of Complementary Care and The Center for Spirituality and Healing at the University of Minnesota; Dr. Dean Ornish, author, Love & Survival and Dr. Dean Ornish's Program for Reversing Heart Disease and Clinical Professor of Medicine, University of California, San Francisco School of Medicine; and Dr. Rachel Naomi Remen, author, Kitchen Table Wisdom: Stories That Heal, cofounder and Medical Director, Commonweal Cancer Help Program and Associate Clinical Professor of Family and Community Medicine, University of California, San Francisco School of Medicine. They are my heroes. They are the true pioneers whose courage and conviction have opened new pathways to healing. All of us are the beneficiaries of their devotion, dedication, wisdom, and hard work. Their Being has been a blessing to both my life and my work. Their spirits strengthened mine, and I am forever grateful.

Introduction

The purpose of this book is to help you find your meaning in your life experiences and to develop a philosophy that is both helpful and hopeful. Some of the aphorisms in this book are new to me, discovered as I researched this book. Other thoughts are old friends that have delighted, inspired, and comforted me for many years. May they connect you with your thoughts in ways that will lead you to strength, peace, and hope.

An old favorite by John W. Gardner is: "Some people strengthen the society just by being the kind of people they are." Those are the people whose stories I have shared in this book. My purpose in storytelling is to awaken your stories. Think of yourself as if you were a glass of soda with bubbles clinging to the sides of the glass and to the bottom. As you read this book, allow your stories to shake loose like those bubbles, rising to the surface of your mind where you can learn from them—and celebrate or discard them.

Ultimately, personal experience is the only valid means we have to understand life—past and present—and to make our choices for the future.

Who looks outside dreams, who looks inside wakes.
—Carl Jung

Winter can be a cozy time—a time to curl up by the fire and listen to music. Winter is traditionally a reflective sort of season—the days are short, the weather can be cold—a good time to sit by the hearth of your mind and look into the fire of your soul.

For me, courage is the overall theme of winter. Outside it is cold and nothing grows. It is dark. There is little out there to sustain us. Winter is the "season" we experience whenever tragedy hits. We are forced to depend on our inner resources. It takes courage to look inside oneself. To what will you awaken if you "look inside?" Looking within is the only path to insights that help to challenge, inspire, and guide us through the tough times.

How do you see courage? A roaring lion? A tall tree? A toddler picking herself up after a fall? A person injecting insulin for the first time? For the hundredth or ten thousandth time?

All art that really draws us to look at it deeply is spiritual.

—Wendy Beckett

Lucy, the delightful Peanuts cartoon character created by Charles Schultz, had a notoriously difficult time catching the baseball. In one hauntingly memorable cartoon, Lucy said, "I was in center field and I saw the ball high in the air. I got under the ball and held my glove in position—confident that I would catch it, when suddenly all my memories of missed catches flooded my mind. I missed the ball. My past got in my eyes."

If you focus your energy on the past, on maintaining your memories of the past, you may not see today's opportunities. Learn from the past but focus on today.

When one door closes, another opens. But we often look so long and so regretfully at the closed door that we cannot see the one that has opened for us.

—Alexander Graham Bell

Never put a period where God has put a comma.
—Gracie Allen

The Menninger Foundation in Topeka, Kansas, is a world famous center for psychiatric care and mental health. Years after the psychiatric hospital was built and its famous programs developed, the observation was made that some mental illness can be prevented. A new center was built on the same campus. It is called the Center for Applied Behavioral Sciences (CABS). At the heart of this organization is this belief: *Your past is not your destiny.*

Begin to weave and God will give you the thread.
—German proverb

A truly amazing thing quite often happens when we undertake a task of great importance. What is necessary for its success begins to appear. We can only guess why. It may be that our focus on the task is so strong that our unconscious mind brings up resources (threads) that had not been in the front of our thinking. It may be that as the project gets underway, other people find out and offer their support. Another explanation is that the new focus and awareness cause you to see threads that may have always been there but were unseen until the task illuminated them.

Perhaps that's how God gives us thread.

The essence of belief is the establishment of a habit.
—C.S. Pierce

If you believe, then you will take action. If we believe in the advice we receive from our health care team, then the next step is to develop healthy habits. When our behavior becomes a habit, it slips easily into our lives.

How do you establish a habit? How do you think you might adopt these habits?

1. Make weekly menus for yourself and keep an ongoing grocery list to be sure you have what you need.
2. Prepare just enough food for each meal. If you don't put it away for lunch the next day right away, leftovers are a temptation to overeat.
3. Place your blood glucose monitor in a location where you will see it and use it—perhaps in your kitchen?
4. Schedule time on your calendar for exercise and make it as convenient and enjoyable as possible.

I use not only all the brains I have, but all I can borrow.

—Woodrow Wilson

How fortunate we are to have all the wonderful advisors whose brain power contributes to our living well with diabetes. We can borrow the brains of an endocrinologist, a dietitian, a certified diabetes educator, nurse, or dietitian, pharmacist, and a psychologist. Another excellent resource that is filled with the latest information on living well with diabetes is the *Diabetes Forecast*, a magazine of the American Diabetes Association (ADA). If you don't get it each month in the mail, join the ADA and you will! It has tips, techniques, guidance, research results, personal stories, and motivation for you.

The greater the obstacle, the more glory in overcoming it.

—Moliere

Each of us has different stories to share about "The greatest obstacle I ever overcame." Do you have one about diabetes? I remember being in Europe for most of a year, thinking I had brought enough insulin with me, and realizing with several months to go that I would run out. That problem was rather easily solved, though. A much greater obstacle came when a doctor I was seeing just before I married, advised me never to have children. He said, "Don't spread your genes around." Overcoming that obstacle involved going to the Mayo Clinic to see a genetic counselor who interviewed both my husband and me about our family history. He gave us real information (positive and hopeful information) on which to make our own decision. His final words to my husband and me were, "Write and tell me if it's a boy or a girl."

Perseverance is not a long race; it is many short races one after another.

—Walter Elliot

Is life with diabetes like that for you? Each day there is a new race to be run, new challenges to face, new questions to be answered. Some days we'd like to "throw in the towel" perhaps. But in our heart-of-hearts, we know that won't lead us where we want to go. So, we lace up our shoes and run another race—and are rightfully proud of ourselves for doing so. You feel better today and better tomorrow because of this dedication.

To reach the port of heaven we must sail,
sometimes with the wind and sometimes against it,
but we must sail, not drift or lie at anchor.
                              —Oliver Wendell Holmes

Where are you today? Where are you in your diabetes management? Are you actively involved in managing your blood sugar levels or are you lying at anchor and ignoring them? What actions can you point to that show you are in motion? Is your attitude focused on living well with diabetes and living life to the fullest, or are you just drifting? This is like a sailor's compass check. You, too, need to keep checking where you are, so you end up where you want to be.

Children are like wet cement. Whatever falls on them makes an impression.

—Haim Ginott

If you were a child when you were developed diabetes, your diagnosis experience had an impact on your attitude toward diabetes. Some of us feel very grateful that we still hold that attitude because it was positive and hopeful. Not everyone's experience is positive. What was yours? Is it still affecting your attitude today? Is that a good thing? Your past does not have to be your destiny unless you want it to be.

Even adults become children in the doctor's office, especially when we are diagnosed with a chronic disease. We all carry memories or fears about diabetes that may have come from our childhood—for example a beloved grandmother having a foot amputation as a complication of diabetes. Look at what formed your first attitudes about diabetes. Is it helping you today?

We have to take reality as it comes to us: there is no good jabbering about what it ought to be like or what we should have expected it to be like.

—C.S. Lewis

Dr. William Menninger of the Menninger Foundation and Clinic wrote a list of the criteria for emotional maturity. First on the list is the ability to deal constructively with reality. Applying that to diabetes we can:

- acknowledge that we have it (no denial)
- avoid the pitfall of "if only" (wishful thinking can obscure reality)
- choose to learn all we can do to manage it
- gather resources to help us
- engage in diabetes management and self-management.

Diabetes is a connection to the real world that we can use to be better than we are. What's really neat is that another reality can emerge: a happy, healthy life.

When we appreciate excellence in others, we make that excellence our own property.

—Voltaire

Going to group classes or group appointments gives you an opportunity to learn how other people with diabetes are managing and coping. In these groups, you can learn helpful and practical techniques for fitting diabetes into your life. You might be surprised at the solution another person has for a problem that has been baffling you. But in addition to the practical lessons, you will be inspired by the brave people who tell you their stories of overcoming challenges and maintaining a positive spirit. You can take that bravery and positive spirit as your own.

When you look for the good in others, you discover the best in yourself.

—Martin Walsh

The only limit to our realization of tomorrow will be our doubts of today. Let us move forward with strong and active faith.

—Franklin D. Roosevelt

In the 1950s, children diagnosed with diabetes were given a 25-year life expectancy. What remarkable faith the parents of those children must have had. No small wonder that they are included in The Greatest Generation.

Upon this gifted age, in its dark hour, falls from the sky a meteoric shower of facts . . . they lie unquestioned, uncombined. Wisdom enough to cure us of our ill is daily spun, but there exists no loom to weave it into fabric.

—Edna St. Vincent Millay

Each of us is a loom. We are surrounded by information on what to eat, how to exercise, why and how we get stressed, and what to do to manage it. It is up to you to pick up threads of courage, wisdom, joy, and faith and to weave them into the fabric of your life.

In the midst of lonely days and dreary nights I have heard an inner voice saying, "Lo, I will be with you."

—Martin Luther King, Jr.

For centuries, the "inner voice" has been written about and revered for the guidance and the mysterious, peaceful assurance it gives believers. We have all known lonely days and dreary nights; some of us even with the profound pain that Dr. King did. Still, we each learn our own lessons.

The words from Dr. King's quote that jump out at me are, "I have heard." He didn't say, "I have read about" or "I have been told about." He said, "I have heard an inner voice."

That inner voice is within you, within me, within all of us. Let us focus on listening for the still, small voice within.

Pause again today. Listen.

There are two ways to live your life. One is as though nothing is a miracle. The other is as though everything is a miracle.

—Albert Einstein

Naturally people have favorite seasons: winter for skiers, spring for gardeners, summer for boaters, fall for hikers. The favorite seasons in our lives might be defined by ages or events. Some we like better than others. But the truly wise person has discovered the value of enjoying it all as Albert Einstein did—everything is a miracle.

Only when you approach life with this perspective do the miracles reveal themselves. The person who grumbles about having to watch a toddler misses the wonder and delight in her discoveries. Those of us with a health challenge may think of the pre-illness days as the best season, but then we are closed to the day-to-day miracles now. I cannot choose to live my life without diabetes. I can choose to see the miracle in blood glucose monitoring, an insulin pump, and the effects of exercise on my body.

Help me to be open to the miracles that surround me.

Always remember that your own resolution to
succeed is more important than anything else.
> —Abraham Lincoln

Your health care professionals want you to do well. Your family, friends, and co-workers want you to do well. As much as you might want to please your health care team or to live up to the expectations of other people, your success is up to you. You will succeed because you want to do it for your self. Think about it.

People with goals succeed because they know where they are going.

—Earl Nightingale

Two important questions to ask yourself are: 1) how much effort are you willing to put in to achieving your goal? 2) how confident are you about achieving your goal? Your responses to these two questions will greatly influence whether or not you succeed. As undeniably important as it is to have a goal, it will just be a statement on a piece of paper unless you put real effort into working on it fueled by your confidence that you can achieve this goal.

Thou dost keep him in perfect peace, whose mind is stayed on thee, because he trusts in thee.

—Isaiah 26:3

For many years, the darkest, most difficult day of my life with diabetes was the day of my annual dilated eye exam. I dreaded going, yet remained faithful to making the appointment, year after year.

I had difficulty because I was afraid that the ophthalmologist would discover eye disease. I didn't want to go blind. Ironically, I thought of not making an appointment . . . but, logic always prevailed. To ignore eye exams meant putting my head in the sand. Denial can be dangerous. Denial of problems does not make them go away. Worse yet, denial could lead to missing the early treatment that could save my eyesight.

As I grew in spirit over the years, fear dissolved into a healthy concern that, miraculously, evolved into peace. The wisdom of the prophet Isaiah helped to direct my focus for each eye appointment.

Most powerful is he who has himself in his own power.

—Seneca

To live well with diabetes you need to be self-aware. You need to know what you want in life. Look at your weaknesses and strengths and decide what to do with them. Remember that dealing with your weakness is often the key to your success. Tap into the positive coach inside you who forgives your shortcomings and encourages your finest efforts.

Go confidently in the direction of your dreams.
Live the life you've imagined.
—Henry David Thoreau

Are you allowing anything to interfere with reaching for your dreams? Sometimes we live as though life were a dress rehearsal—it isn't. Don't put your life on hold because of temporary setbacks. Get busy realizing the dreams you hold dear for they are unlikely to materialize without your effort. See the Big Picture. Pick up your palette and do something every day to help paint your life as you want it to be.

The point is that our true nature is not some ideal that we have to live up to. It's who we are right now, and that's what we can make friends with and celebrate.

—Pema Chödrön

While prayer can be defined as talking to God, meditation is listening to God. Connecting with the spirit requires listening. Robert Esbjornson, retired religion professor, talks of a meditative way of paying attention while you are reading, writing, conversing— even eating and exercising—that opens you to the world of your own soul.

Meditative listening to find deeper meaning opens us to messages we may miss in conversation. So often we hear the words but not the wisdom. Bob's advice is: "Listen for something that touches your soul."

The next step is meditative writing. You write your response to what you are reading or hearing. The writing can be directed to yourself or to God. Meditative writing can help clarify your thoughts and beliefs. This active way of meditating keeps you aware so your reading and conversing can bear spiritual fruit.

Listen. . . .

An individual's sense of personal control determines his fate.
—Martin Seligman, *Learned Optimism*

After 27 years of imprisonment, Nelson Mandela was asked how it felt to be free. His response was: I have always been free. Some people see diabetes as taking away their freedom. They see the struggle for control as a tug-of-war between them and the disease.

At the diagnosis of diabetes when I was ten years old, I drew the proverbial line in the sand, and let it be known that I would be in control. Hospitalized nearly two weeks, I had to have blood drawn each morning for a blood glucose. The staff found it difficult to find my veins, and the whole procedure became very painful and difficult. One morning I made a promise to myself that I would get married in a state that did not require a blood test. There would be one blood test I could control. Fifteen years later one more blood test didn't matter, but when I needed to believe that I could be in control of my life, I was.

Today's mighty oak is just yesterday's nut that held its ground.

—Author unknown

A spiritual winter can blow into town in any month. The tell-tale signs of "frost" include despairing statements like these:

- "I am working out regularly, and I still don't have the toned body I want."
- "I'm monitoring blood glucose levels, making the best decisions I can, and I still have highs and lows."

Without predictable outcomes, how do you keep going day after day after day? Being faithful to your values, not living for results. Is it possible that:

- Faith is more important than outcomes?
- Frustration can teach me patience?
- My steadfast determination will inspire others?
- Disappointment actually strengthens me?
- Success, when it comes, will be even sweeter because of my struggles?
- Success may have an entirely new and deeper meaning?

It is possible. So, I keep going.

I am not afraid of storms, for I am learning how to sail my ship.

—Louisa May Alcott

One of the gifts we can receive from diabetes is self-confidence. Until we experience difficulty in life, we really don't know how we will respond.

Like sailing, diabetes requires specific skills. Nutrition education helps us to navigate through grocery stores and restaurants. Exercise education leads us to explore what type, how much, how often, and the very important question: what do I enjoy? The "meds" in diabetes education include "medication" to address physical need and "meditation" to meet mental and spiritual needs.

To sail the ship of diabetes successfully we need to know the physical information. Equally important is psychological, social, and spiritual hardiness to take on any of the storms that life presents.

When we discover that we can manage diabetes, then we gain a boost of self-confidence. The blessing in this self-confidence is that it does carry over to other life challenges. We've handled one; we can handle another.

Courage is fear that has said its prayers.
—Dorothy Bernard

After my father died, I seized every story that might tell me something about him. I was given a prayer book that he had received from the Methodist Church. I read it repeatedly, wondering what disappointments it had helped him to bear. Had he taken it to Europe when he served in World War II? Pondered it while he built his law practice?

I learned more about his family when I was given his grandmother's Bible. As I leafed through the tattered pages, I saw that she had read with frequency the books that I love—especially the Psalms. In the back of her Bible was a tithing covenant that she signed in 1929. A widow with four young sons, she committed to a ten-percent tithe to the church at the beginning of the Great Depression. These stories were woven into the fabric of my life as I sought the courage to live with the challenges that life was presenting to me.

Nothing endures but personal qualities.
—Walt Whitman

In his poem *What Endures*, Walt Whitman reminded me that nothing outside of me is as great as the qualities that lie within me. This process of self-reflection is at the heart of the power of poetry and is, I believe, its purpose.

The libraries in our communities hold many books of poetry. Now, when poetry is no longer our school assignment, perhaps we can return to poetry on purpose and discover . . . ourselves.

Even if snow covered the world completely, the sun could melt it with a glance.

—Rumi

Winter is a metaphor. It can represent difficulties, loneliness, darkness, cold, and despair. We all are vulnerable to a winter spirit. Spiritual winters can hit us any time, even on a bright, sunny day in July.

However, when a dreary spirit comes on us on a cold, blustery, cloudy day in January, we feel that blast of winter doubly hard. Mental health experts talk about seasonal affective disorder (SAD) causing depression in the winter because of the short days and the lack of sunlight. An antidote is to increase the light in your surroundings. I have at least one extra lamp turned on in our living room all winter. Perhaps that helps prevent the physical disorder.

My spiritual light comes from music, laughter, poetry, and prayer . . . beaming light into the dark corners of my heart.

If you are patient in one moment of anger, you will escape a hundred days of sorrow.

—Chinese proverb

Elisabeth Kübler-Ross identified a process that people experience when they lose a loved one. The process is similar when you lose a dream—disbelief, anger, sadness, denial, alternating hopefulness and hopelessness, and finally, acceptance.

Psychologists can help people get from anger to acceptance. Many people find their own path. A mother told me about her young daughter with diabetes who gets fed up every once in awhile with having to have injections of insulin. Her path to healing began when she made a small pile of used, plastic syringes with the needles clipped off. She stamped her feet again and again on the syringes, venting her anger, and shedding her tears until she felt better.

How do you vent your anger? Hitting a golf ball? Punching a pillow? Engaging in strenuous physical activity? Writing out your thoughts, and then, making a ceremony of tearing up the paper?

Anger is a natural feeling. It is neither good nor bad; it just is. How we handle anger makes it a destructive force or an empowering one. The last time you were angry, what did you choose to do?

The last of the human freedoms—to choose one's attitude in any given set of circumstances—is to choose one's own way.

—Victor Frankl

Following a presentation to a group of people with diabetes, I was approached by a delightful, older gentleman. With twinkling eyes and a huge smile, he said, "My pappy always said, 'Ya gotta have an attitude of gratitude!'" He told me that his father had been one of the pioneers in insulin therapy, receiving insulin in the 1920s. Now, in the 1980s, his father was alive because of the miracle of insulin and ALIVE because he chose to be. He had chosen an attitude of gratitude.

Each day each of us is faced with choosing what our attitude is going to be. We certainly can't always choose our circumstances. Victor Frankl was in a Nazi concentration camp during World War II. He lost everything. He could make no choices about his life. But he discovered that he could choose his attitude. He chose to be hopeful. Not only did he survive, he was alive with his sanity and compassion intact.

Real courage is risking something you have to keep on living with, real courage is risking something that might force you to rethink your thoughts and suffer change and stretch consciousness. Real courage is risking one's clichés.

—Tom Robbins
Another Roadside Attraction

Philosophers tell us that human growth has its roots in pain. Those who do not experience growth get stuck in a philosophy like this one: "Life's a bummer; then you die." For others, challenges like a chronic disease can become the vehicles that carry them on a journey of self-discovery and growth.

Between these extremes of "Life is difficult" and "Difficulties help me grow" is a middle ground where our philosophy might be: "This is the way life is, so I'll make the best of it."

The famous figure skater Scott Hamilton had cancer. I saw him skate following his surgery and recovery. He gave a dazzling, energetic, beautiful performance. His inspiring spirit is evident in this statement of his: The only disability in life is a bad attitude.

The heart eats food from every companion; the head receives nourishment from every piece of knowledge.

—Rumi

I read a newspaper article one winter about the need for winter "comfort foods." Psychologists remind us that eating for comfort can lead to obesity . . . and high blood sugars for people with diabetes. Consider the "comfort foods" that nourish your spirit. One of my favorites is a bouquet of daisies. Fresh flowers in February are so delightfully unexpected that they jolt me into noticing them. Daisies invariably lift my spirits.

Comfort comes from other sources: a talk with a soul mate, a gathering of friends, the familiarity of place (home, club, place of worship), the familiarity of routine (humdrum as routine is to us, at times, there is comfort in its changelessness). And comfort comes from knowing that the "still small voice" within us will always be there. These are, indeed, nourishment for the spirit—giving us comfort.

What lifts you out of a wintry spirit? What are your spirit's comfort foods?

My friends have made the story of my life . . .
turned my limitations into beautiful privileges,
and enabled me to walk serene and happy.
—Helen Keller

How generous of Helen Keller to give credit to her friends for turning her limitations into privileges. We, none of us, can make it alone in this world, especially when we are challenged by illness. But it was Miss Keller herself who made the story of her life by redefining her limitations. In her remarkable life not only did she overcome blindness and deafness to communicate with the world around her, but she also became a famous author and lecturer.

She teaches by her example the lesson expressed by British philosopher Aldous Huxley: "Experience is not what happens to you; it's what you do with what happens to you." The decisions, choices, and actions that Helen Keller made enabled her to walk serene and happy.

The universe is full of magical things, patiently waiting for our wits to grow sharper.
—Eden Phillpotts

A question frequently explored by both health care professionals and people who have diabetes is: "Why do people find it difficult to follow their diabetes regimen?" Although people with diabetes know how to manage diabetes, quite often they don't act on that knowledge.

When do you find it difficult to follow the regimen of meal plan, regular exercise, medication-taking, and stress management? What are the barriers?

I have gathered some insights over the years about these barriers, such as a lack of support, a poor self-image, poor coping mechanisms, feelings of powerlessness, bad habits, hopelessness, and the fact that the disease never goes away. All these can lead to falling off the wagon or a reluctance to even get on the wagon.

Being aware of your difficulties is an important step in setting and reaching your goals.

Behold I do not give lectures or a little charity.
When I give, I give myself.

—Walt Whitman

Feelings of isolation and loneliness provoke some of our darkest hours. People who don't have diabetes cannot understand what it is like to live with diabetes. Even in the midst of loving family and caring friends, we can feel lonely. We can feel isolated even though we are surrounded by caring health care professionals.

Support groups can fill that need for us. A support group is a place where wisdom dwells, and courage fuels discussion. Generally, humor warms the discussion and softens the rough edges of feelings. Confidentiality wraps her arms around the group, and respect brightens every gathering. Whether people sit around a table or in rows of chairs, they always gather around the campfire of the human heart. A support group provides a place where people can tell their stories to listeners who care, but don't judge or offer advice. Each of us just listens and cares . . . and probably understands.

Consider attending or forming a support group of people trying to live well with diabetes.

One of the things I learned the hard way was it does not pay to get discouraged. Keeping busy and making optimism a way of life can restore your faith in yourself.

—Lucille Ball

Andrea Meade Lawrence was an Olympic alpine skier. In one of her runs down a mountain during Olympic competition, she hit a flag and fell. Without missing a beat, she got up and continued down the mountain. She won the gold medal.

What do you suppose her thoughts were when she hit the flag? "Oh darn. I blew it." That thought could have led her to give up. The fact that she kept going suggests that her thoughts were ones of courage, determination, and faith. She believed she could make it—and she did.

What are your thoughts when you hit a flag in your life, such as experiencing an unexpectedly high or low blood sugar? What helps you keep going? What are the thoughts that help you get up when you're down?

Live each season as it passes; breathe the air, drink the drink, taste the fruit, and resign yourself to the influences of each.

—Henry David Thoreau

Winter in the north and summer in the south are sometimes thought of as seasons that need to be endured until the next season arrives and the weather isn't so severe. Happy (and wise) are those who find things to enjoy in all seasons . . . including each of the seasons of life from childhood through old age. Savor, don't just endure.

We are the hero of our own story.
—Mary McCarthy

Joseph Campbell studied heroes. From the Bible, from Greek mythology, from virtually every known culture, Campbell studied what he called the "hero's journey." The journey begins with a crisis, which Campbell referred to as the call to adventure. We've each received that call. We have a choice about whether or not we will answer. To ignore or deny the call is to risk losing an opportunity for learning and growth. When we answer the call, we find the experience to be transforming.

Plug your experience with diabetes into this description of the hero's journey. Did your diabetes begin as a crisis? Did you choose to deny it for awhile? If you did accept the call, what have you learned and how have you grown? How have you been transformed?

Be strong and of good courage; be not frightened,
neither be dismayed; the Lord your God is with you
wherever you go.

—Joshua 1:9

Diabetes introduced me to the "what ifs." It's a torturous game that most of us play but few of us win . . . unless you call "winning" the insight that there will always be more questions than answers.

After my son was born, I experienced a new level of concerns over what would happen to my family if I were to experience serious complications of diabetes. I wondered what it would mean to be a blind mother . . . what if . . . what if . . . .

My son was a toddler. I was spending a lot of time reading to him. What if I couldn't read to my child? The response to that question gave me the peace that I sought. What if my son would read to me, and this experience would strengthen his character? I could begin to receive peace from these thoughts because I value character development.

I continued to receive peace when I thought through the roles that God and I play. I do the best I can to manage my diabetes on a daily basis. He takes all my worries and replaces them with peace . . . if I believe.

I gain strength, courage, and confidence by every experience in which I must stop and look fear in the face.

—Eleanor Roosevelt

Winter can symbolize struggle and difficulties of life . . . such as diabetes. The diagnosis experience is often a wintry time in the lives of all the people affected: you, your family members, and your friends. Anger, fear, resentment, and depression are common responses to the diagnosis. And so is courage.

Courage keeps us going as we travel through our difficulties, exploring our strengths, learning all the lessons that life has to teach.

What is there to see in the fearful face of diabetes? Complications of blindness, kidney failure, and nerve damage? Strength, courage, and confidence came out of the DCCT and UKPDS, research studies that showed a modest improvement in A1C levels cut the risk of these complications in half or more.

We need courage, not to face the complications as if they were inevitable, but courage to live the healthy life that makes them preventable.

Whatsoever things are true, whatsoever things are honest, whatsoever things are just, whatsoever things are pure, whatsoever things are lovely, whatsoever things are of good report . . . think on these things.

—Philippians 4:8

As we move through life, there are changing circumstances—from technologies to social trends. This is fertile ground for discovering new lessons about Life.

Computers have introduced quite a few changes to our lives and can help us understand an important lesson about personal choice and responsibility. We have more power when we view ourselves as the programmer, not as the program acting out someone else's design.

We can actually program each day by the goals we set. Sometimes our goals get redirected because Life has other plans for the day. But if we begin each day with goals, at least we'll start in a direction of our choosing.

We are all sculptors of ourselves.
—Henry David Thoreau

One day a man observed his neighbor in the backyard standing by a huge rock, with hammer and chisel in hand. The man walked over to his neighbor and asked what he was doing.

"Oh, I thought I'd try my hand at sculpting," was the reply.

The man said to his neighbor, "But you have no training, no experience. You're crazy!" and he left that day on vacation. When he returned two weeks later, he was astounded to see in his neighbor's backyard a perfect sculpture of an elephant.

He went directly to his neighbor and demanded, "How'd you do that?!"

The humble neighbor shrugged his shoulders and responded, "I don't know, I just chipped away everything that didn't look like an elephant."

Oh, words are action good enough, if they're the right words.

—D. H. Lawrence

Consider your use of certain words and what thoughts and feelings arise from them. Do you "test" your blood glucose or do you "monitor" it? Some of you may say it's the same thing. Others will see the difference as significant.

Testing implies pass or fail. The word *test* is judgmental. Since people do not like to fail or feel like a failure, some (out of fear of failure) may not check their blood glucose. However, if you say and think *monitor*, there is a different meaning and feeling. To monitor is to seek information. The data collected is used for decision-making, not judging. Your thoughts about blood glucose monitoring can make it a burden or a blessing. Compare these thoughts:

1. As if age, weight, income, and IQ were not enough, blood glucose results give us another set of numbers by which we can judge ourselves . . . or be judged.
2. Blood glucose monitoring provides me with information that helps me to be in control of my life. I can have greater safety and comfort when I know where my blood glucose level is.

We can choose our thoughts. Are yours helpful?

You cannot prevent the birds of unhappiness from flying overhead, but you can prevent them from building a nest in your hair.

—Chinese proverb

Thoughts come into our minds, but we do not have to let them stay! Although it is important to know about diabetes complications and how to prevent them, it can be dangerous to focus too much attention on them.

One danger is that we become so fearful of complications we miss the joy and fulfillment that can be ours today. Another danger is that people fear an event so much that they begin to expect it to happen, and may help cause it to happen. Psychologists explain this by saying that we move in the direction of our most dominant thought.

The birds of happiness and the birds of unhappiness are all around us. Which will you invite to build a nest in your hair? When frightening thoughts appear, we can choose what to do with them. One of the best ways I know of sending them on their way is to replace them with life-affirming thoughts. I focus on hope and all the values that keep me motivated to manage diabetes.

Health and cheerfulness mutually beget each other.

—Joseph Addison

Be grateful for whatever comes, because each has been sent as a guide from beyond.

—Rumi

What are your values that motivate you to take up the daily challenges involved with the management of diabetes? Although I can readily tick off the values in my life (such as love for family, desire to have the energy to do my work well, the very basic desire to feel well), I appreciate holding in my heart more poetic expressions of those values. Because I do not consider myself poetic, I am always appreciative of those who are.

Such a poet was a soldier in the Persian Gulf. His lovely, thought-provoking comment was, "I'm ready to fight . . . but I'm here for the sunsets."

My thought in response to his comment was, "Aren't we all?"

Although I do not like the metaphor of war/violence/fighting, I know that I'm ready to take on whatever challenge that I must. However, I'm not looking for struggles to overcome. I'm looking for beautiful sunsets to enjoy.

That's the poetic reason that I poke my fingers, take insulin, eat nutritiously, and exercise regularly.

I love sunsets.

Difficulties strengthen the mind, as labor does the body.

—Seneca

"Into each life some rain must fall," says Henry Wadsworth Longfellow's poem *The Rainy Day*. I ask questions: What do you mean by rain? A sprinkle? A gentle, steady rain? Heavy winds and hail? A hurricane? A light rain makes flowers bloom and grass grow. Heavy winds, hail, and a hurricane do damage.

So, what was Longfellow trying to say? That rain must fall so grass and flowers can grow? Or that rain, symbolic of life's challenges, is part of everyone's life? For me it says life has problems to help us learn to cope and solve problems. Rain helps us appreciate the sun ever the more because we have known darkness.

Robert Fulghum says in *Uh-Oh: Some Observations from Both Sides of the Refrigerator Door*, "but, a lump in the oatmeal, a lump in the throat, and a lump in the breast are not the same lump." That's the sort of discernment I need when I consider the rain that falls in my life. I hope that I can be philosophical about the smaller problems. "Some rain" is good for my garden, and challenges help me grow.

Look not mournfully into the Past. It comes not
back again. Wisely improve the Present. It is thine.
Go forth to meet the shadowy Future, without fear.
—Henry Wadsworth Longfellow

Sometimes we create our own winters of despair. Overindulgence in food is perhaps the most common challenge for people with diabetes. People who have an alcohol problem can give up alcohol completely. People with diabetes have to continue to eat. Many people with diabetes actually plan for an occasional overindulgence and "weather" the experience well.

Many people, however, report that they are filled with remorse, regret, and guilt following an experience of overeating. Because thoughts create feelings, one might speculate that the thoughts in this instance would include shame, self-criticism, and hopelessness. These thoughts can lead to more overeating when people just give up and stop trying to get back in control of their lives.

Let us approach these times of winter with compassion for ourselves. Now is the moment to take action. Let the past go.

Traveler, there are no paths. Paths are made by walking.

—Australian Aboriginal saying

One woman's ingenious response to chemotherapy made the experience manageable . . . even beautifully meaningful. The woman wrote to her children and her friends. She asked them to send her something that was meaningful to them. She also asked for the story of the meaning in the object. She planned to return each to its owner after she had taken it to the chemotherapy sessions. This plan was a way to keep herself distracted from the chemotherapy and to remind herself of all her loved ones— her reason for wanting to live.

It worked better than she could have predicted. At each appointment, she set out the treasures sent by friends and family. As she set each one down, she told the story behind it. Sometimes a member of her family or a friend was with her. The nurse administering the drugs got so involved that sometimes she would start telling the story behind one of the treasures to the guest. The woman had wanted the items to remind her of her loved ones. She didn't realize how much love was there to share.

Sunshine is delicious, rain is refreshing, wind braces up, snow is exhilarating; there is no such thing as bad weather, only different kinds of good weather.
—John Ruskin

It seems that retirement—like life—is what you make it. A woman who had looked forward to retirement was surprised to find that once retired, she found life boring. She had no energy because she no longer had something to look forward to daily.

Then she discovered an exciting and meaningful project. She collects various flowers and weeds and makes them into works of art. In spring, summer, and fall, she collects materials. In winter she dries, arranges, and frames them to sell at craft fairs. This simple project has had an enormous impact on her attitude. Once again she is excited, enthusiastic, and happy. She would tell you that there are no bad seasons in life, only different kinds of seasons.

Retirement is the summer joy of finding things you like to do, the fall wisdom to do them, the winter courage to try new things, and the spring faith to keep saying "Yes."

*God, grant me serenity to accept the things I
cannot change, courage to change the things I can,
and wisdom to know the difference.*
—Reinhold Niebuhr

This *Serenity Prayer* is world famous. Many of us know the prayer, and yet we forget what it means when we get busy. It is only through reflection, our inward journey, that we remain aware of our vast resources. If we have known serenity at any point in our life, then serenity is one of our resources . . . however deeply buried it may be.

Something like the loss of a job can make people feel backed into a corner. They have to do something, but worry consumes them. When they can let go of the worry, they experience the serenity that will help them take the next step and the next.

Think of a time when you felt a total calm that could be described with the word serenity. Close your eyes and recapture that moment. Then, apply that serenity to something in your life that you cannot change. Has diabetes backed you into a corner? Or do you have serenity in your corner backing you up?

We cannot change the way the world is, but by opening ourselves to the world as it is, we may find that gentleness, decency, and bravery are available—not only to us, but to all human beings.
—Chögyam Trungpa

Continuing to think about Niebuhr's Serenity Prayer, what memories come to you when you think of courage? I remember being a skinny 12 year old about to give my first abdominal injection of insulin. I didn't want to do it. That was back in the days when we used steel needles and glass syringes. Shots were painful, and I did not want to push one of those "nails" into my tender midsection.

No less than two doctors coached me. I finally pushed the needle into the pinch of skin, only to have it come right out the other side of the pinch. I quickly glanced up to catch the most horrified expressions on the faces of the doctors. Suddenly, I felt very brave.

Every experience we have ever had with courage becomes a resource for us in the future. Courage begets courage. It builds upon itself.

When you reread a classic, you do not see more in the book than you did before; you see more in you than there was before.

—Clifton Fadiman

The third spiritual quality in Niebuhr's prayer is wisdom. It is wisdom that keeps us returning to the well of our inner resources to draw on past experiences, the lessons learned, the dreams yet to be realized, and the faith that we really do have all the resources we will ever need.

Inspiration and intuition team up to connect our plain, everyday experiences to the wisdom that lies deep within us. When this happens, we typically have one of those Aha! moments. When the staff of a clinic in Wisconsin invited me to speak at their annual meeting, I asked whether they had a theme. They told me: The Wizard of Oz. This Aha! immediately connected me with the SERENITY (heart) of Tin Man, the COURAGE of Lion, and the WISDOM (brains) of Scarecrow.

I enjoyed the movie *The Wizard of Oz* when I was a child. I enjoy it year after year. I continue to marvel at how much meaning this adventure film has. This quote helped me to understand how this could be.

The *Wizard of Oz* provides many rich metaphors. The Wizard himself is a metaphor for the magic bullet—the sure cure that so many of us seek, convinced that an answer to our questions exists outside of us. But, ultimately, he was a scam artist. He used Dorothy and her friends to get rid of the Wicked Witch of the West but did not—because he could not—deliver on his promise to return Dorothy and Toto to Kansas.

Dorothy herself had the power to return to Kansas. She had the ruby red slippers and the mantra, "There's no place like home." Lyrics to the song "Tin Man" by the band *America* reinforce the idea that answers are found inside of us, not outside. Each of us has the wisdom we need.

Oz never did give nothin' to the Tin Man that he didn't, didn't already have.

The happy result of the Wizard's scam tactics was to put the requests back on the people doing the asking, which resulted in their empowerment—they discovered their own resources!

It is tempting to sleepwalk through life. To tell half-truths, listen half-way, be half-asleep, drive with half-attention . . . . Wake up!

—SARK

When a friend of mine who is characteristically optimistic and upbeat was depressed, he told me that he actually welcomes feeling "down." He explained that these depressions don't last. The lesson they bring is that they make him aware of feeling. "I am grateful that I can feel," he told me. "I may not celebrate feeling down the way I celebrate joy, but both joy and despair are needed to make me whole."

Instead of having the rug pulled out from under your feet, learn to dance on a shifting carpet.
—Thomas Crum

Remember how you feel when an irritating noise, flashing light, or body ache suddenly stops? Perhaps you experience a calm, relaxed state. Awareness of that calm is similar to "being present in the moment." This expression is used by people who engage in mindful meditation.

A calm, relaxed state is best for spiritual communication. The "still, small voice within" can be heard better when inner turmoil is quieted.

A psychologist friend said he recommends to clients that they close their eyes and imagine a large gunnysack outside the room in which they meditate. He suggests dropping each concern into the sack where it can be retrieved later. Our concerns need to be dealt with, but meditation requires a quiet mind, a peaceful soul.

Just to be is a blessing.
Just to live is holy.

—Rabbi Abraham Heschel

When we have nothing, we learn a lot about ourselves . . . and about life. We learn what we value, what we really need, and who we really are. Without distractions like money, power, position (even a job), we can focus on what we do have. This is a crash course in values clarification.

Diabetes has the power to drive the same process.

Just when we feel we've been deprived of the good that life offers (desserts? the lifestyle of a couch potato?), we realize that the promise of the good life is an empty promise, and we re-evaluate the meaning of "good life."

What is included in your definition of the good life? What values and beliefs do you live by? Are there simple pleasures that delight you? Are you engaged in meaningful work (volunteer or otherwise)? Do you give of yourself to help others?

There is a turning around we must accomplish.
—Buddha

A father who had lost his 14-month-old son to heart disease commented that there is no getting over the loss of a child but that a "new normal" evolves. In this new normal, there can be laughter and joy. He had not believed that normal joy could be part of his life anymore. He said that working on a charity event to raise money for the local children's hospital made his new normal brighter.

After a while, life with a chronic disease evolves to a new normal. Diabetes can be viewed initially as a series of losses: the loss of the former self, the loss of the previous lifestyle, the loss of a dream. However, a new normal evolves, and we can see our new self as stronger and our new lifestyle as healthier, New dreams emerge that can be more deeply meaningful and precious.

Barn's burnt down, now I can see the moon.

—Masahide

A dear friend of mine shared a story with me about her experience with kidney dialysis. Several times a week she had to be hooked up to a dialysis machine. To say it was a task she did not enjoy would be a great understatement. My friend struggled with her feelings—gratitude that she could be kept alive through dialysis, yet resentful of this largely unpleasant experience that took her away from meaningful activity.

One day the nurse who worked with her told my friend that she was studying to become a naturalized citizen of the United States. From that time on, whenever my friend had dialysis, she quizzed the nurse about American policy and citizenship. The time passed quickly, and my friend experienced the great reward of knowing that she was helping someone.

All the world's a stage.

—William Shakespeare

Shakespeare said that we are actors on the world's stage. We play many roles. "Diabetic" does not describe who I am, but I believe that word does describe one of the roles I play in life.

In the theatre, actors play their roles only when they step onto a physical stage. In life, we are "on stage" every moment of every day. We play numerous roles at the same time, but always we play our diabetic role.

There are certain roles that I enjoy more than others. I like my roles as wife, mother, and educator. Actually, it is because of the roles I enjoy that I work at doing the diabetes role well. I want to continue enjoying my current roles, and I want to be healthy so that I can experience the future role of a happy, healthy retiree.

Never change a winning game. Always change a losing one.

—Bill Tilden, world-class tennis player
who had diabetes

In the book *Gung Ho* by Kenneth Blanchard and Sheldon Bowles, I read a marvelous analogy. "Running a business from numbers is like playing basketball while watching the scoreboard instead of the ball." Eureka! I immediately saw the application in diabetes. Managing diabetes by focusing on blood glucose numbers reduces diabetes self-management to a numbers game and ignores the bigger picture—the game of life and the person who is playing it.

Blanchard and Bowles advise business people to look after the basics if they want success, and the first basic is the person. Is the person happy? It's the same in diabetes. Is the person enjoying life? Is the person experiencing a (self-defined) fulfilling life? Is the person coping well? How is the person? When the person is doing well, the numbers will reflect that.

Results! Why, man, I have gotten a lot of results.
I know several thousand things that won't work.
—Thomas A. Edison

I often hear people say that having diabetes in and of itself is not so bad. What is tough are all the management tasks—daily, even hourly—carrying out the appropriate eating, exercising, and monitoring. Life with diabetes is a never-ending juggling act. And if, from time to time, one of the "balls" gets dropped, it is not because the juggler is noncompliant, that is, uncooperative. Balls get dropped because constant, never-ending juggling is tiring, tedious, and difficult.

The greatest strength is gentleness.
> —American Indian proverb

Eleanor's story is a story of love, courage, wisdom, and faith. Eleanor is my mother. I have told this story on three continents to thousands of people.

I was diagnosed with diabetes in 1957 just ten months after my father died. Mother was a 39-year-old widow with her second great challenge: a little girl with a chronic disease, diabetes. When I asked my mother what diabetes meant, she smiled and enthusiastically told me, "Diabetes means that we are going to learn so much about good nutrition. It means that we're going to live such a healthy lifestyle, the whole family will benefit because you have diabetes. And you will always be a stronger, more self-disciplined person because you have diabetes."

She set me on a healthy path. That positive attitude gave me strength to cope with diabetes. Nineteen years later I drew strength from what she taught me when our son was seriously injured. Before we knew the lasting impact of his injury, I knew it would make him strong. Her legacy is one of love and wisdom and faith.

Thank you, Eleanor.

Wisdom is a tree of life to those who embrace her;
happy are those who hold her tightly.

—Proverbs 3:18

The diagnosis of a chronic disease can cast a shadow over the future. People sometimes respond to their diagnosis by putting future plans on hold.

As we approached the year 2000, I was aware that people historically (or hysterically?) view a new millennium as potentially the end of the world. Fearful questions arise. One of our pastors gave a sermon on the new millennium. His conclusion was: It's time to plant a tree.

When I was diagnosed with diabetes as a child, people in our small community commented to one another that I would not live to be 21 years old. Forty-seven years after diagnosis, I am enjoying the fruits of a healthy life. I'm grateful that my mother planted a tree . . . the tree of life.

Luck may sometimes help; work always does.
—Folklore

Being resilient is an important quality in life. We frequently observe it in nature. I have seen robins rebuild nests after it was demolished by a blizzard. Flowers beaten flat to the ground by wind and driving rain find a way to stand up again with the return of gentler breezes and sunshine.

There is a spirit of resiliency in the human soul that amazes some, escapes others, and inspires those who are willing to invest in it. Diabetes is filled with examples because living positively with diabetes requires that we be resilient.

Diabetes does not go away. Neither is it easily managed. Many variables affect blood glucose levels from hormones to stress. If only we could quit diabetes the way we can quit a job. But we can't, so we make a decision about that in which we will invest.

What is the return on an investment in self-pity? What is the return on an investment in blame, denial, or anger?

I am resilient when I invest in such blue chip stocks as courage, faith, joy, and wisdom. The return on that investment is a richer, fuller life, including living well with diabetes . . . or any challenge.

When we overcome our pain (physical or emotional), we are immediately connected to an elite of humankind, people who have also risen above pain. There are many. Here are statements from two of these special people.

The marvelous richness of human experience would lose something of rewarding joy if there were no limitations to overcome. The hilltop hour would not be so wonderful if there were no dark valleys to traverse.

—Helen Keller

I have learned that success is to be measured not so much by the position that one has reached in life, as by the obstacles which one has overcome while trying to succeed.

—Booker T. Washington

No man is an island.

—John Donne

Rituals give us ways to address life events, giving the events meaning and the rituals purpose. In the early 1970s, in the aftermath of the Vietnam war, many people wore the names of soldiers missing in action around their wrists to lend support. The intent was to wear the ID bracelet until the soldier was found.

It was 1976 when our baby was born . . . and seriously injured because of a hospital mistake. He needed to remain hospitalized after I was released. I cut the plastic hospital ID off my wrist, but I left the second hospital ID on . . . it was John's.

I went to the hospital each day and spent the entire day there, nursing, bathing, enjoying my baby. At night I returned home. Twenty-seven days after John was born, we brought him home. That evening as we sat at the kitchen table, I took the kitchen shears and quietly cut the ID from my wrist. Our little MIA was home at last.

With all the heartache and concern over John's injury, I had been helped by wearing his ID. I felt connected to the many people whose concerns were similar though far greater. I drew on their strength. I hope they received some of mine.

Since every failure is a lesson, every challenge an opportunity, and every joy a triumph, it's hard to go wrong.

—Michael Addison Reed

Joseph Campbell studied heroes from ancient literature, including the Bible and Greek mythology. Campbell pointed out the huge dilemma that the human race faces. We want to have strength without hard work. We want to be heroic but not have to suffer. But, growth only comes as we travel through pain. It is our trials that transform us into heroes.

When diabetes enters our lives, we can refuse to answer the call to adventure, at great risk to our health and well-being. Or we can choose to accept the call with all the challenges and problems in it.

Another aspect of the hero's journey is that the hero has an advisor who helps guide him through the "snakes" and "dragons" along the way. The advisor for those of us traveling with diabetes is our diabetes health care team.

Don't leave on your journey without them.

The lack of knowledge is darker than the night.
—African saying

The mother of a friend of mine was diagnosed with diabetes. I was quite young and made the assumption that my friend's mother was making the same lifestyle changes that I was, learning much of the same information for living well with diabetes.

Many years later, I returned to my hometown for a funeral. I was surprised when I saw my friend's mother and realized that she had had a leg amputated. I was stunned when I heard her ask, as sandwiches were being passed to her, "Is there any sugar in these?"

She had never learned the basics about diabetes. She didn't know about which foods are converted into glucose. What happened?

Let each of us serve to guide people to the American Diabetes Association, to a diabetes educator, to education—the beacon of light that is life.

If you surrender to the wind, you can ride it.
—Toni Morrison

Surrender is very difficult for most of us to do. We want to be in control. But when we feel in need of help, the idea of surrender becomes appealing . . . if we feel trust and faith in the person or entity to which we surrender.

When we were very small children, the fortunate among us had parents who were worthy of our trust . . . people to whom we could surrender when we were getting in over our heads. That's why I like the image of God as a Heavenly Father . . . completely worthy of my trust.

Surrender to the wind symbolizes the ultimate spiritual act: trusting the unseen. If the wind symbolizes the spirit, what would it mean to you to ride it? I can imagine being taken through the tree tops, into a bird's nest, and landing gently on a flower petal. I try to imagine the myriad places that this wind could take me.

I surrender.

This is the true joy in life, the being used for a
purpose recognized by yourself as a mighty one; . . .
the being a force of Nature instead of a feverish
selfish little clod of ailments and grievances
complaining that the world will not devote itself to
making you happy.

—Bernard Shaw

Stories of how people have courageously over-come their difficulties are a great source of inspiration. We all seek to celebrate a triumph of the human spirit.

Marilyn Hamilton fell from a hang glider and ended up paralyzed from the waist down. She complained one day to her hang-gliding friends that wheelchairs were like steel dinosaurs: heavy, awkward, and ugly. They got together to design a wheelchair using the lightweight metal used for hang gliders.

The result was the Quickie wheelchair . . . and a successful new business venture. Marilyn designed the wheelchairs to have vibrant colors. She says: "If you can't stand up, stand out."

That is spirit. Her story is a triumph and an inspiration.

It is a sort of splendid torch which I have got hold of for a moment, and I want to make it burn as brightly as possible before handing it on to future generations.

—Bernard Shaw

People who inspire us can be (and often are) an ongoing source of inspiration. My mother always has been.

One Thanksgiving she invited our entire extended family: my married sisters' in-law, the aunts, uncles, and cousins . . . lots of people. Because I lived out of town, I couldn't be there to help with anything except the last minute details. Concerned for my mother, I asked her, "Why do you work so hard?"

With joy in her face, she responded: "Because I'm so thankful that I can."

Every tomorrow has two handles. We can take hold of it with the handle of anxiety or the handle of faith.

—H.W. Beecher

Anxiety is common to all of us. Beecher's comment makes it seem as though we have simply to choose between anxiety and faith. But grasping hold of the handle of faith is not easy, it is not a "simple" choice.

In fact, it is a choice that we make many times, through many tomorrows. How often have I chosen to have faith, to let go and let God, only to find myself wrestling back the control for anxieties that I really want no part of? Life is very ironic at times.

Let us explore our choices . . . again. Let us choose life.

Life is either a daring adventure or nothing.
—Helen Keller

This brings an image of covered wagons rumbling across the plains. People moving with all their belongings to a place they've never been . . . places no one's been. For most of us, "daring adventure" invites thoughts of physical challenges—biking across the state, scaling tall mountains, or swimming the English Channel.

But by the courageous, enthusiastic way Helen Keller lived despite being blind and deaf, she demands that we take a deeper look at what we call a daring adventure. Blindness makes an adventure out of the simplest tasks, like getting dressed or cooking a meal.

Whatever the destination, we have to face our fears of the unknown. We have to go inside to find the courage it takes—whether we are changing careers, taking the trip of a lifetime, injecting insulin, or writing a difficult letter to a friend.

What have your most daring adventures been—physically, emotionally, mentally, spiritually? Have you ever had the experience of slipping your hand into God's and saying, "Yes. Whatever—wherever. Count me in."

To laugh often and much; to win the respect of intelligent people and the affection of children; to earn the appreciation of honest critics and endure the betrayal of false friends; to appreciate beauty; to find the best in others; to leave the world a bit better, whether by a healthy child, a garden patch or a redeemed social condition; to know that even one life has breathed easier because you have lived. This is to have succeeded.

—Ralph Waldo Emerson

Check-up time. Are you living as fully as you really want to? If not, what can you do to live more fully? Make a plan and do it. Now.

Prepare to be amazed.

It would be very good if we would wake up before we die.

—Old Hindu saying

Great art hangs in museums. Great art is heard in concert halls and celebrated in theatres. There is, in addition, a great art that resides within each of us. Henry David Thoreau called it the highest of arts: the art of living. People who practice this art are not artists in the usual sense. They are people who, through the nobility of their lives, have affected what Thoreau called the quality of the day.

We can affect the quality of the day for ourselves and others . . . turning dark to light . . . fear to courage . . . frustration to patience . . . loneliness to joy. Our words are music just as surely as our lives paint a picture. From our hearts, through our words and actions, we create the beauty of kindness, patience, harmony, and hope.

When I see someone engaged in an act of kindness, I am watching a great artist creating a masterpiece, affecting the quality of the day for everyone.

Be careful the environment you choose for it will shape you; be careful the friends you choose for you will become like them.

—W. Clement Stone

Do you have more drinking buddies or exercise partners? Look at your calendar. How have you spent most of your weekends? Where do you generally go and with whom? Think again about how you're choosing to live.

In the depth of winter I finally learned that within me there lay an invincible summer.

—Albert Camus

Life brings many winters. My friend lost her teenaged daughter in a car accident. She found strength from Camus' words because she could believe that her daughter, for all eternity, would remain in the spring of her life. A disease is one of life's winters. The force that keeps you going through the darkest hours of the harshest winter is Hope.

Wise living may be less in acquiring good habits
than in acquiring as few habits as possible.
—Eric Hoffer

Habits are automatic behavior. Habits allow you not to think, not to feel. They also rob you of the new experience that you could have in this moment. If you had no habits, every action would be a conscious choice. That could result in healthier behavior for your mind and body. It could also make you very tired to have to think through every action. Still, it might be worth observing your habits for a couple of days. It's the only way to see those habits that are not useful or helpful to you.

A man too busy to take care of his health is like a mechanic too busy to care for his tools.

—Spanish proverb

So what excuses do you use for not having regular, health-promoting activity in your daily schedule? What happens to tools that are not well-maintained? What happens to your health without maintenance? What are you doing today? How about a 15-minute walk after dinner?

In nature, nothing is perfect and everything is perfect. Trees can be contorted, bent in weird ways, and still they're beautiful.

—Alice Walker

Just for today consider each person you encounter as perfect. Study him and her and find the ways in which they are beautiful. Help them to see their own beauty, and you will begin to see more of yours reflected in the eyes of your new friends. This is how to boost your own spirit.

The most beautiful thing we can experience is the mystery.

—Albert Einstein

Near the end of each winter when I have looked so long at the frozen world, I begin to think about the mystery and miracle that we will experience when spring arrives. The sun touches seemingly dead branches, and the tree responds with a "Yes!" to life. It sends forth tiny buds containing green leaves that surprise me each year with their freshness, lacy beauty, and remarkable spirit. This never fails to awaken and inspire my spirit, too.

The mystery of life—how does it happen? Again, the physical season mimics the spiritual—or is it the spiritual that mimics the physical?

*We could never learn to be brave and patient if
there were only joy in the world.*
                                    —Helen Keller

All of us have hurts. Many of us experience
tragedy. These become part of our story, part of who
we are. But we can actively seek healing—which on
the soul level is acceptance of what has happened and
love of who we are right now.

The miracle is that we can be whole again. I have
my healing stories and have heard the healing stories
of many people. Some have nothing to do with diabetes but all deal with the human dimension of hurting, finding hope, and healing. When we choose to
seek healing, we are involved in what Thoreau called
"the art of living."

Diabetes cannot be cured, yet. Some diseases can
be cured, but even then, the person who had the disease may not be healed. While we join hands in working for a cure, may we also offer our hands to one
another to promote healing.

When I was nine years old, my father died unexpectedly of a heart attack. Three weeks after I turned ten, I was diagnosed with diabetes. These life events inspired some deep thinking that may be unusual for children that age. Although I still thought about childhood games and goals, I asked questions about the meaning of life . . . questions more common to middle age.

I remember a prayer that I said every night:

I do not ask a truce
With life's incessant pain,
But school my lips, Lord,
Not to complain.
I do not ask for peace
From life's constant sorrow,
But, give me the courage, Lord,
To face tomorrow.

The prayer never struck me as being morbid or sad. Saying it helped me feel strong by connecting me to the source of my strength. At the age of ten, I was a wise little old lady. I knew that life was tough . . . and, still, joyful.

People are like stained glass windows; they sparkle and shine when the sun is out, but when the darkness sets in, their true beauty is revealed only if there is a Light within.

—Elisabeth Kubler-Ross

Poets, philosophers, and theologians talk about the importance of inner light to illuminate the spiritual path. You must find the light that is within you, and learn to use it. That's why people engage in meditation and thinking about the self: to explore and define the source of that inner light and to experience it each day.

*Where there is hope, there is life, where there is life,
there is possibility, and where there is possibility,
change can occur.*

—Jesse Jackson

The DCCT and the UKPDS studies gave us proof that we can prevent or slow down complications, such as blindness, kidney failure, and nerve damage—giving us all hope for healthier futures. So, why aren't people more interested in learning about the diabetes management that led to the positive outcomes? Maybe it seems like a lot of work. Maybe they don't think you can enjoy life and manage diabetes intensively.

We need to see the POSSIBILITIES. Diabetes educators can expand your view. Explain your concerns about intensive management. Learn the latest techniques to manage your diabetes in any situation. You might be surprised when you discuss how these techniques can support your lifestyle. See new possibilities for yourself.

With HOPE and lots of POSSIBILITIES, you can make the changes you choose to make.

Imagination is more important than knowledge because knowledge is limited.

—Albert Einstein

An endocrinologist looked into my eyes 20 years ago and said, "You'll need treatment within the year." Although I am grateful for retinopathy laser treatments, I had never needed them and didn't want them. I had no plan but to have faith and remain open.

Then I attended a class called Creative Visualization and Mental Imagery. The lecturer said that the mind can heal when we visualize the hurting part as healed . . . not healing, but healed and whole. I decided to visualize my retinas as perfectly healthy, with no microaneurysms. I found a photograph of a healthy retina and taped it on a door. I looked at it everyday and imaged that beautiful retina as my own.

At the next appointment, my endocrinologist said the problem was gone. How is that explained? I'd started using a glucose monitor and getting A1C tests. Maybe it is because I had good diabetes tools that I have never developed serious eye disease. Perhaps it is because there is a mind/body connection that I tapped into. Perhaps . . . both?

You can combine survival and celebration.
—Chögyam Trungpa

Laura's Garden commemorates the life of a little girl who died following a horse riding accident. The garden, at the elementary school, was built by her family, friends, principal, and teachers, a community seeking healing. At the dedication, her pastor said, "The question is not *where* is God? The question is *when* is God? And, the when is now." We saw God's and Laura's spirit in:

- Statements of love from her parents, sister, and aunt
- A poem read by a family friend
- A song written as though from Laura, thanking people for her garden
- Essays written by classmates, read by the school social worker
- The large group of children and adults gathered to celebrate Laura and her garden
- The trees, plants, flowers, waterfall, pond, and bridge
- The tiny new butterflies released at the end of the ceremony

I go to this place of beauty to remember my parents, my nephew, my son's college roommate, aunts, uncles, and friends.

Always search for your innermost nature in those you are with.

—Rumi

In the 1980s, I served on the board of an inner city hospital in Minneapolis. We decided to merge with another hospital, hoping we could be financially stronger together. The interesting part is that we merged a Christian and a Jewish hospital. So everyone in our new hospital would feel nurtured, the board mandated a Spiritual Focus Committee. We all felt blessed by this experience as we learned about one another's traditions and worked together for our patients, our hospital, and our community.

A Christian chaplain and a Jewish rabbi dedicated our All-Faiths Chapel. The rabbi gave the benediction: "May we continue to respect our differences and love what we share." As with all great truths, that statement can apply to all communities and could lead to world peace.

I saw another application—in chronic disease. There is a "community" of people with chronic diseases. There are differences among arthritis, lupus, asthma, heart disease, and diabetes. Our challenges may be different, but we share the spiritual values of love, hope, peace, wisdom, and joy.

Hope is the pillar of the world.

—African proverb

HOPE is the very cornerstone of life. But for some, hope can be wishful thinking. People can hope for things, experiences, and results. Hope in this context is a verb. For others, hope can be the faith on which the foundation of their life is built. They have hope, no matter what circumstances they face. Hope in this context is a noun.

How do you use the word hope? How much wishful thinking do you do? Listen for the word hope when you speak. What evidence do you find that hope is the foundation of your life?

Are you hoping for a good life or do you have hope that you will?

*The people who make a difference are not the ones
with the credentials, but the ones with the concern.*
—Max Lucado

Friends, family members, co-workers, fellow
church-goers, and the many people we encounter in
our daily lives make a difference when they show their
concern for us. They are part of our health care team
because they promote our health as human beings. Do
these people in your life know that you have diabetes?
If not, why?

In the PBS show *Amazing Grace*, Bill Moyers interviewed country singer Johnny Cash about the song's power. Cash recalled having sung *Amazing Grace* to prison inmates. He said, "For the three minutes that song is sung, everyone's free."

Singer Judy Collins, who also recorded *Amazing Grace*, told Moyers that when she sings it, there is a "mystical territory" between the song and the audience. Finding a power all its own, the song heals.

I recall a difficult time in my life when I played Judy Collins' *Amazing Grace* every day. For the minutes that I listened to her singing, I experienced the freedom that Johnny Cash referred to and the healing that Judy Collins recognized. I felt connected to the thousands of people who have listened to or sung this beautiful hymn and, taking spiritual refreshment from the song, have turned to meet adversity with courage and grace.

Seek the music that nourishes your spirit.

In a Positive Psychology class at Harvard Medical School, we learned the biological benefits of responding to humor. The many different lab results showed that the powerful benefits of laughter can be totaled up as a powerful increase in immune system activity and a decrease in stress hormones. The next slide in this lecture put the issue into perspective:

Humor can be dissected as a frog can, but the thing dies in the process and the innards are discouraging to any but the pure scientist.

—E.B. White

Live in a perpetual great astonishment.
—Theodore Roethke

As thinking beings, we develop a philosophy of life whether we realize it or not. What is yours? It may only show up in your attitude toward others or toward what happens to you.

In developing a philosophy of your own, you might take some tips from two famous philosophers.

It is better to travel hopefully than it is to arrive.
—Robert Louis Stevenson

Strong hope is a much greater stimulant of life than any single realized joy could be.
—Friedrich Nietzsche

You don't live in a world all alone. Your brothers are here too.

—Albert Schweitzer

Dr. Hans Selye, a Montreal physician, when he was alive was an international expert on stress. When asked "How do you manage stress?" he said, "There are three pieces of advice that I follow.

First, decide if you are a turtle or a race horse and respect that.

Second, set your own goals.

He said the third was the most important, "Give of yourself to help others." He called this altruistic egotism and said, "When we help others, we help ourselves."

The rainstorm is not personal, and yet we get
personally wet.

—Werner Erhard

Apparently Selye was also a believer in the now common guidance that we should learn to reframe our troubling or negative thoughts. This method acknowledges that our thoughts create our feelings. And our feelings have strong influence over what we do—or will try to do.

Said Selye: "Nothing erases unpleasant thoughts more effectively than concentrating on pleasant ones." This is a powerful tool for good health that you can start using right now.

A kind word is like a Spring day.

—Russian proverb

Choice is a critical aspect of living well with challenges like diabetes. We choose our behaviors and our attitudes. We choose how responsibly we will take action on the information we get from our health care team and from daily blood glucose monitoring. We choose the thoughts that will help to make diabetes self-management an onerous burden or an opportunity for good health and personal growth.

I have a poster in my office that reminds me of the most basic choice of all, the choice of life itself. Reflect on your choices and on these words:

Before you this day there is set good and evil, life and death . . . .Choose life.

—Deuteronomy 30:19

In late March of 1998, a tornado ravaged southern Minnesota. More than a mile wide, the tornado uprooted trees and shattered homes into splinters. My friend and mentor, Robert Esbjornson, lost nearly everything. His computer was sucked into the angry sky. A treasured painting was stolen by the unrelenting force of the wind. His bed was reduced to its metal frame. Momentos of a 45-year marriage—gone. The arboretum in front of his picture window was now treeless.

As he walked through the rubble and surveyed the damage and devastation, he said he could hear a sort of music in his head. When he paused to listen, he realized that he was hearing bits of Psalms going through his head. A habit of reading a Psalm each day was providing him with strength, peace, and comfort.

> When I thought, "My foot slips," thy steadfast
>   love, O Lord, held me up.
> When the cares of my heart are many, thy
>   consolations cheer my soul.
>
> —Psalm 94:18,19

It is wise to furnish one's mind well. When it's all you have left, you want a rich treasury.

May the Footprints we leave behind
Show that we've walked in Kindness
Toward the earth and every living thing.

This lovely thought was inspired by American Indian philosophy. It is an example of how we can transcend or rise above the many, momentary problems of daily life.

Some days we get so concerned about dusty footprints on a newly waxed floor that we miss the bigger picture . . . of life. Pause today to see above the daily challenges and ponder the footprints you are leaving.

Only an open mind still has room for new knowledge.

—Robert Fulghum

One Sunday morning as I listened to the children in our Sunday School program sing, I received the gift of an awakening to a new thought. The children were moving their hands through the air as if their hands were boats going through waves. The words to the song were: "With Christ in my vessel, I can smile at the storm."

In that very instant, I saw vessels to mean blood vessels, not boats. I experienced a peace that told me no matter what the future holds, I don't need to worry.

I cannot possibly know the details of what that means. I can't "know" that I will never develop blood vessel complications. But, at a far deeper level of understanding and life, I can and I do know that I will be fine. What amazing peace there is in that.

APRIL 9

All my life through, the new sights of Nature made me rejoice like a child.
—Marie Curie

Spring has a magical beauty that inspires thoughts of new beginnings. The lacy, light, yet brilliant green of new leaves is a thrilling sight each year. The earth's agenda to bring about new life inspires me to examine what I am doing to rejuvenate my life.

I will busy myself, along with Mother Earth, at the tasks of life. What the earth does naturally, she has reminded me to do intentionally—self-care. I will recommit to the goals of good nutrition and invigorating exercise. I will take my "meds" (medications) and I will do my "meds" (meditations).

In mindfully attending to the health of my body, mind, and spirit, I am engaged in true self-care. The Earth and I are one.

Exposure to beauty can awaken the memory of beauty that resides in the soul. So, too, can hearing or reading wisdom awaken that quality within us. Consider the wisdom in this beautiful Talmudic saying:

> *Just as the hand held in front of the eye obscures the tallest of mountains, so can the stresses of everyday life keep us from seeing the awe, the wonder, and the mystery there is in the world.*

What real or metaphoric "hand" might you have in front of your eyes? Name the stresses that currently obscure your vision.

What names can you give to the awe, wonder, and mystery that surround you?

Painted prayers are found in India where women are responsible for these visual petitions to the gods. Traditionally, these painted prayers ask for health and well-being.

Consider what your painted prayer would be. Instead of words, what would a prayer of pictures include? Would you have people in your picture? What would their faces look like if you were praying for spiritual qualities like peace, hope, joy, and love?

If you were praying for healing and wholeness, what symbols might you use in your painted prayer? What colors would you choose? Red for enthusiasm, love, and compassion? Green for peace? Blue for wisdom? Yellow for joy?

Consider your painted prayer. Paint it if you have that gift. But at least, close your eyes and paint your prayer in your mind.

Work of sight is done. Now do heart work on the pictures within you.

—Rainer Maria Rilke

APRIL 12

A United States senator told Mother Teresa that no matter how hard she worked, millions of people would die. Her task was hopeless. Mother Teresa's remarkable response was:

God does not require that I be successful. He asks that I be faithful.

Managing diabetes is not only a daily task, it requires hourly attention . . . if only a glance at your watch to see when the next meal, monitoring, or exercise will occur.

The rewards most people seek include daily good health and the reasonable hope of avoiding serious long-term complications. There is a reward at a deeper level. It is integrity of the spirit—the very spirit that Mother Teresa spoke of.

You can experience integrity of the spirit when you follow healthy attitudes and behaviors with no guarantees of a reward. That's diabetes management. That's life.

Life is full of important tasks that we work at without being guaranteed success: parenting, marriage, jobs, friendships. Although there is no guarantee, there is a reasonable expectation that the harder we work, the better we will do. On my most frustrating days, when blood sugars defy me, I realize that I may not be successful, but I can be faithful.

APRIL 13

Self-efficacy—the belief that we are capable—
is regarded as one of the primary indicators that we will
do well with a disease that requires self-management,
a disease like diabetes. If people believe they can perform the tasks that manage their disease, they are more
likely to perform them.

Whereas I do believe that, I also believe at a
deeper level that I need more than self-confidence. I
need God confidence—the faith and belief that I am
not alone.

And that He who is with me has the power to
spin the galaxies. Such is my faith in God.

*Trust in him at all times, O people; pour out your
heart before him; God is a refuge for us.*
—Psalm 62:8

Lo, I am with you always, to the close of the age.
—Matthew 28:20

Sometimes our light goes out but is blown into flame by an encounter with another human being. Each of us owes the deepest thanks to those who have kindled this inner light.

—Albert Schweitzer

We can have our inner lights kindled by people whom we know and by people whom we will never meet. We nourish hope by what we read and hear. Then, in moments of quiet reflection we reconnect with that wisdom. Here are some of my favorites. What are yours?

To give without any reward, or any notice, has a special quality of its own.

—Anne Morrow Lindbergh

The future belongs to those who believe in the beauty of their dreams.

—Eleanor Roosevelt

None are so old as those who have outlived enthusiasm.

—Henry David Thoreau

We do not possess our home, our children, or even our own body. They are only given to us for a short while to treat with care and respect.

—Buddha

When my son was born, an IV solution burned away the skin, tissue, veins, and nerves from knee to foot. The scars always draw comments. We helped him with responses for simple questions and rude ones. As a junior, he was getting his ankles taped before football. A young physician was telling the boys, "I had four years of college after college to become a doctor." Then he saw John's leg, "What happened to you?"

John's response, "Oh, some guy with four years of college after college made a mistake." I wish he had told the young physician we never sued.

His team visited a children's hospital. John kneeled by a little boy in a wheelchair. The boy said, "I love playin' baseball, but they say I won't walk the way I used to." John rolled up his pant leg as the little boy rolled up his pajama leg. They shared their scars, their stories, and their strength. None of us will ever be quite the same.

Don't fight forces; use them.

—Buckminster Fuller

David, the humble shepherd boy, conquered the evil giant, Goliath, using a slingshot and a well-placed smooth stone. Christians and Jews alike celebrate this Biblical hero.

David's single greatest attribute was his faith. He knew how small he was in comparison to Goliath. He surely would have felt more confident leading an army to stand with him against his foe. With no army and only a slingshot for a weapon, David relied upon the greatest power in the universe: God.

What are the "Goliaths" you face in life? Is diabetes one of them? How does faith play a role? It was faith that led David to pick up his slingshot and use it.

If David's tool was a slingshot, then maybe our basic tool is a blood glucose meter. Diabetes can seem like such a huge obstacle that hopelessness becomes the real Goliath. It takes enormous faith to pick up our tools and use them.

There are years that ask questions and years that answer.

—Zora Neale Hurston

The year that you were first diagnosed with diabetes brought many questions. What does this mean for me? How will diabetes affect my life—my relationships, work, and family; the hobbies and recreation I enjoy; the goals I have; and the overall enjoyment and fulfillment I find in life. How have the years since answered those questions?

If you have faith the size of a mustard seed, you will say to this mountain, "Move from here to there," and it will move; and nothing will be impossible for you.

—Matthew 17: 20–21

When John was six years old, he found a baby robin had fallen from its nest. In Minnesota we fill a cardboard box with grass and leaves, put the bird in it, and feed it oatmeal and skim milk through a medicine dropper.

One look at this robin told me it couldn't make it. Its feathers were still wet. It was too premature to live. Gently, I told John that we would do our best. My son leaped into the air exclaiming: "His name is Oscar." I cringed. It would be so much harder when the bird died now that it had a name. At bedtime, John remembered Oscar in his prayers. I cringed again, but we prayed.

Oscar made it.

Before the healthy robin flew away, he perched next to our garage. My neighbor took a photo. That photograph is still on the door of our refrigerator. The photo of Oscar reminds us all of how little we know—knowledge isn't really what is important. Faith is.

APRIL 19

The diagnosis of diabetes, or any chronic disease, brings lots of questions. Why me? Why now? What does the future hold? Health care professionals can project—some even predict—but no one can know enough to answer these questions.

Living comfortably with unanswerable questions requires faith. Elie Wiesel, one of the best known Jewish writers, survived Auschwitz and wrote:

> *Heaven is the place where questions and answers become one.*

A similar thought is expressed in the Christian tradition by the apostle Paul:

> *For now I see in a mirror dimly, but then face to face. Now I know in part; then I shall understand fully, even as I have been fully understood.*
> —1 Corinthians 13:12

Where do you turn for comfort with your unanswerable questions?

The golden moments in the stream of life rush past us and we see nothing but sand; the angels come to visit us, and we only know them when they are gone.

—George Eliot

Do you believe in angels? On topics such as this, I listen to my heart to make my own decision, but my head also listens to people whom I respect. My friend Bob Esbjornson refers to angels as "messengers of El," the Hebraic idea of angel. The book of Hebrews has a statement about angels: "Do not neglect to show hospitality to strangers, for thereby some have entertained angels unawares." I have heard and read that statement many times over the years. I have wondered at its meaning. My own response has been, "But, I'm busy, and my house is a mess." I have only looked at the meaning literally, to mean people coming into my house.

Bob refers to messages as angels, too. The messengers can be the ideas in a book or a movie or lecture. He refers to authors as strangers to whom he opened his mind, and he was hospitable to the message. He said, "It's a matter of being hospitable to strangers, to people with ideas that are unfamiliar to me but somehow connect with ideas at home in my mind."

For he will give his angels charge of you to guard you in all your ways. On their hands they will bear you up, lest you dash your foot against a stone.
—Psalm 91:11–12

A favorite print that my great-aunt had in her home showed two small children standing on a rickety, old bridge over a river. The little boy was leaning over precariously as if to retrieve a shiny stone. Unbeknownst to either child, an angel had her finger through the belt loop on the back of his trousers.

Although that is both a lovely and a comforting thought, I believe there is an important issue of self-responsibility, of stewardship. I do believe in angels, but I also believe that I am expected to do the best I can to act responsibly and not demand that angels protect me when I am acting irresponsibly. This belief leads me to monitor my blood glucose levels often so that I can drive a car safely, exercise with plenty of "fuel," and keep my blood sugars in a range that will not harm my blood vessels.

Consider where you are on the angel issue as well as on your responsibility to yourself.

Time heals all wounds.

—Anonymous

After our son was injured, two experiences led to my healing eight years later. The first was a sermon by a pastor who has a severely handicapped son. He said he literally shook his fist at God and asked, "Where were you?!" (I never dreamed pastors got angry at God! That helped my feelings of guilt.) He said that he felt God's response was: "I was there . . . grieving with you."

The second was when I spoke at a risk management conference. I was invited because the physician in charge knew about my son's injury and that we had never sued. He wanted me to share our story.

At the end of my presentation, I said, "There's one thing I don't understand. The hospital never apologized to my husband and me. Are hospitals so afraid of culpability that they cannot be human?" It was a rhetorical question. A man came up and said, "I know the hospital you're speaking of. I work there but wasn't there when your son was born. I'm eight years late, but on behalf of the hospital, I apologize to you and your husband." Tears of healing streamed down his face and mine.

My father-in-law immigrated from Norway. He met and married my mother-in-law, and they had the first of three children. When World War II broke out, my father-in-law was drafted. When he returned, he wanted to be a carpenter but was told that he needed the union's permission. The union refused because he was inexperienced and, at age 34, too old.

My in-laws discussed the situation, and my father-in-law began to cry at not being able to provide for his family. My mother-in-law gathered her composure and sang a hymn that gave her strength.

> Oh, what peace we often forfeit; Oh, what needless pain we bear.
> All because we do not carry everything to God in prayer.

When she finished, she squared her shoulders and said: "You go back to the union and tell them all the experience you do have. Then, you tell them that if you can fight for your country at age 34, you can certainly become a carpenter's apprentice." He went to the union, and the rest, as they say, is history. We attended the celebration honoring his 50 years in the carpenter's union.

Faith has many faces . . . my mother-in-law's is one of them.

Faith is a bird
Which feels the light
And sings in the dark
Before the dawn.

—Anonymous

Energy, for a variety of reasons, can become low in people who have diabetes. Low blood sugars can leave us feeling virtually lifeless. Beyond physical energy, it is spiritual energy that keeps us going on our darkest days through the roughest places on our walk.

What carbohydrate is to a low blood sugar, inspiring words are to the spirit.

They who wait for the Lord shall renew their
strength,
they shall mount up with wings like eagles,
they shall run and not be weary,
they shall walk and not faint.

—Isaiah 40:31

Reading and rereading great literature is important because each reading can bring new meaning. The Psalms were my great-grandmother's favorite. I have her Bible, and the Psalms are tattered and torn from her rereading of this sacred and meaningful text. One of her four sons, my great-uncle Andrew, was killed in World War I. The Psalms may be where she found comfort, strength, and peace.

When my son had surgery at the age of four, I was very concerned about the anesthesia. My concern centered around a mistaken dosage . . . too much anesthesia.

I found peace in Psalm 121:

The Lord will keep your going out and your coming in from this time forward and for evermore.

We are not human beings having a spiritual experience. We are spiritual beings having a human experience.

—Pierre Teilhard de Chardin

When people experience Life's toughest times, quite often they turn to the power they recognize as greater than they are. Making this connection or re-connection is life transforming . . . the proverbial blessing in adversity.

Some people describe their experience as one of using the spiritual to help them transcend the reality of their pain. Others say that their painful experiences, as unwelcome as these are, help them to focus on what they truly value—spiritual values.

So, the question seems to be: Are we transcending reality or ascending to reality?

*The only tyrant I accept in this world is the still
small voice within me.*

—Mahatma Gandhi

Great stress is created when we feel pushed to respond to the commands and demands of others. At times we may even feel that our lives are controlled by tyrants. We can experience tyranny at work, at home, at medical appointments . . . Sorting through the various demands, we must decide for ourselves what is important.

"The Torah wants me to stay healthy," says Rabbi Ave Boruch Hollander. In an article in the February 1997 *Diabetes Forecast* magazine, Hollander goes on to say, "That's why I take my diabetes regimen as seriously as I take my religion." An orthodox Jew, Hollander believes that the Torah, the law of Moses, relates to every part of his life—including diabetes and diet. He explained: "Torah tells us that one good deed brings another, and that one sin brings another. When I make one good food choice, odds are that I will make another good food choice. And, when I make a poor food choice, I usually follow it with another poor food choice."

Hollander describes his interweaving of religion and health this way: "Torah asks us to live in the real world. And food and health, and certainly diabetes, are in the real world."

And what is his real world motivation? "I would like to be around to dance at my children's grandchildren's weddings."

Incline your ear, and come to me; hear, that your soul may live.

—Isaiah 55:3

Isaiah's ancient advice holds great insight into the nature of our spiritual life. The most obvious meaning in this passage is that as we read and listen to God's Word, we will be nourished spiritually. We will be spiritually alive.

I also understand in Isaiah's words that we are to listen to our hearts . . . where God resides. We are, in fact, to seek God everywhere and as we seek, we shall find.. With the intent of finding God, I can incline my ear to a flower . . . and find Him.

The voice of God is always speaking to us and always trying to get our attention. But His voice is a "still, small voice," and we must at least slow down in order to listen.

—Eugenia Price

Within you, there exists a stillness and sanctuary to which you can retreat at any time and be yourself.

—Siddhartha

The kingdom of God is within you.

—Luke 17:21

God calls us away from the tumult of the world, so
we may focus our lives on things that are lasting.
In God's presence we see our lives more clearly;
the broken pieces are put back together. God calls
us out of loneliness into a life of community.
Worshipping together, caring about one another,
we find out what it means to be truly human.
                              —Pastor Terry Morehouse

A humble, informal church service in a rural setting began with this prayer that clearly explained why we were together on a "retreat." Community is a key component to healthy living. In community we know that we are not alone. We can receive support and give support.

Diabetes is one of many examples of the brokenness and isolation in the world. Support groups, local hospitals, clinics, and places of worship provide us the opportunity to create community and heal the brokenness. And, when we help one another to heal, we discover what it means to be truly human. We realize that we are not broken; we are whole.

Spirit comes from a Greek word that can also mean breath or wind. We do not see wind any more than we see the spirit. But everywhere we can see the evidence that they exist.

Leaves swirl, branches sway—although we don't see the wind, we see what it does. What evidence exists for the spirit?

Page through the book of your life. Where have you seen, heard, or experienced any of these fruits of the spirit?

Love
Joy
Peace
Patience
Kindness
Goodness
Faithfulness
Gentleness
Self-Control
—Galatians 5:22

Do you have experiences or stories that make each of these fruits real?

i thank You God for most this amazing
day:for the leaping greenly spirits of trees
and a blue true dream of sky;and for everything
which is natural which is infinite which is yes
> —e.e. cummings

Each of us has a string of pearls . . . in our hearts. These "pearls" are the beautiful moments we've experienced thus far in life. These are moments that become memories that will:

Uplift
  Enliven
    Gladden
      Soften
        Inspire
          Guide

There are plenty of baubles, bangles, and beads in life . . . and only a few true gems. Close your eyes and see your string of pearls. Name the gems—by person, by place, by experience, by gift of the spirit. Whether or not you wear jewelry . . . wear your spiritual string of pearls.

Let everything that breathes praise the Lord!
—Psalm 150:6

In the Hebrew language, there is no word for "thank you." When thanks appear in Hebrew writing, the word used is the Hebrew word for praise. What connection do you find between thanks and praise?

What is an "attitude of gratitude?"

Writer C. S. Lewis described praise as "inner health made audible." What does inner health mean to you? What does it look like? Is it healthy organs? A healthy mind? A healthy spirit? What causes it to become "audible?"

Does its audible expression mean singing? Shouting? Laughing? Speaking in a whisper?

May we see not only with our two eyes
But with our one eye which is our heart.

—Black Elk

Sometimes anguish is caused by a misunderstanding. Years ago I was in a Bible study. During our small group discussion, a woman blurted out: "I just can't be thankful for all circumstances!" She was referring to a scripture passage. But she misunderstood it.

Our group discussion leader calmly and gently spoke. (She had lost her five-year-old son to leukemia.) Beth said, "The actual passage reads: "Give thanks in all circumstances, not for all circumstances."

As Beth's words sank in, we watched the weight of the world lift from the woman's shoulders. It pays to ask questions. Sincere seeking is not disrespectful. The rewards can be great.

God changes not what is in a people, until they change what is in themselves.

—The Koran

Diabetes is a chronic disease—there is no cure for it. How we live with that fact directly affects the quality of our lives. And, although a cure is not yet found, healing is possible, and, in fact, healing can greatly enhance our quality of life. Cure is a physical act. Healing is spiritual.

Consider where you are spiritually. Are you on a healing path? What signs in your life tell you that you are on a healing path? A healing path might include: engaging in meditation, praying, discussing feelings, having a support network, journal-keeping, acknowledging the need to heal, and actively seeking healing.

Signposts along the healing path can include feelings of peace, faith, hope, and courage; an attitude of acceptance rather than resignation; and the belief in your heart-of-hearts that your experience with diabetes has given you insights that you value.

What are they?

At my church, I facilitate a group of people who have chronic health challenges. Some have diabetes. It is not our individual health challenge that brings us together. It is our desire for wholeness. We recognize that physical ailments cannot always be cured, but that healing is always a possibility . . . and we actively seek that healing.

I wrote this prayer for the group. What additions or changes would you make so that it would speak for you?

Dear Lord,

We come before you seeking wholeness. Heal us as it is your will to do so. If total physical healing is not your Plan, then we pray for the grace and strength to accept our challenges.

Grant us health and healing of our minds and spirits. May we have wisdom to live faithfully, love to give to all with whom we interact, joy in the many gifts You provide us daily, and peace forever in our hearts.

Thank you, gracious Lord.

Amen.

Grief hollows us out that we may hold more joy.
—Kahlil Gibran

The spiritual side of life is where we explore and find courage, joy, wisdom, faith, steadfastness, hope, and peace—among other spiritual qualities. Where does the following thought lead you? Agree or disagree, but know what you think and why you think it.

Fear, stress, pain, and loss are our truest gifts because it is their presence that calls forth the spiritual qualities from deep within us.

What is your philosophy? What is your belief about suffering? How do you heal?

Exercise has the effect of defusing anger and rage, fear and anxiety. Like music, it soothes the savage in us that lies so close to the surface. It is the ultimate tranquilizer.

—George A. Sheehan, MD

When I do my workout, I almost always include a brisk 30- to 40-minute walk for the aerobic part. As I walk, I pray. When I make the petition "Create in me a clean heart and renew within me a right spirit," I ask for clean arteries, veins, and capillaries. I ask that my heart be cleansed physically, emotionally, and spiritually.

As I ask for the renewal of a right spirit, I ponder recent events in my life. Identifying my shortcomings and weaknesses, I ask for strength.

Then, I listen.

Talking is the easy part. Listening is hard. Sometimes the still, small voice is very, very quiet.

Youth never despairs, for it is still in harmony with the Divine.

—Alexandre Dumas

When our son was in second grade, he had a Sunday School teacher who assigned scripture to be memorized each week. One Sunday evening after checking the assignment sheet affixed to our refrigerator door, I told John that the week's memory verse was *Trust in God.*

"Oh, good!" he said enthusiastically, "that's easy." My eyes immediately met my husband's as we non-verbally communicated our understanding that it is not easy to trust. My next thought was that John meant that three words are easy to memorize. My lasting belief is that childlike faith does include an ease in trusting God. It is adulthood that creates dis-ease or disharmony through disappointments that have not been reconciled.

For years I taught first grade Sunday School. I presented the weekly lesson. But I learned as much as I taught. The children provided the lasting lesson of trust. We don't have to lose our childlike faith.

The best way with music, I imagine, is not to bring the forces of our intellect to bear upon it, but to be still and let it work on that part of us for whose sake it exists.

—George MacDonald

Music therapy is now a major course of study offered at colleges. Schools are keying into what intuition has told us for centuries. Music has potent power to heal. In 1988, I gave the keynote address for the American Association of Diabetes Educators. I predicted that music would be part of our spiritual approach to healing. I jokingly predicted that diabetes educators might need signed, informed consent forms to play music as powerful as that of Neil Diamond.

Use musical therapy based on your unique needs and desires. Consider today the music that you like. Do you have several types that appeal to you for different reasons? Is there one that helps you manage stress, another that revitalizes your spirit, calms, energizes, or. . . . What are the ways you use music?

My planet was blown up with all my clothes in it,
you see. I didn't realize I'd be coming to a party.
—Douglas Adams
Life, the Universe, and Everything

Diabetes is an unwelcome intruder in the lives of people who already have challenges with which they must cope. "Why me?" is a common question. "Why?" is also a common question found in the Psalms.

In his book, *Psalms for Sojourners*, James Limburg points us to some interesting thoughts about the Psalms. The question "Why?" is directed to God; the question is never answered. But the Psalms do not end with questions. They move to affirmations, and, in nearly all of them, the Psalms end with words of praise.

As we travel our journey with diabetes, we find many questions to explore. The fortunate among us find life-affirming experiences and fellow travelers that lift us when the questions have no answers. We are truly blessed if we can end our journey with words of praise.

Life is what we make it, always has been, always will be.

—Grandma Moses

Focus on a health outcome that you want. It may be weight loss, physical endurance, or flexibility; it may be improved A1Cs. Your hoped-for outcome may be a mental or spiritual goal of feeling in control of your life or being at peace. Name the outcome you want to focus on today.

Then review the steps you have taken in the past in your attempts to achieve this outcome. Think especially of the outcomes that have eluded you. Is today's approach similar to what you've done in the past?

If so, maybe that's the problem.

If you always do what you always did,
you will always get what you always got.

—Moms Mabley

We shall not cease from exploration;
And the end of all exploring will be to arrive where we
    started
And know the place for the first time.

—T. S. Eliot

Development continues for all of our lifetime. We learn more about ourselves and the world each time we encounter one another. The process of gaining insight seems to require us to explore, reflect, apply, and evaluate.

Each review of familiar places and experiences presents us with a new perspective. Thus it is that we can "arrive where we started and know the place for the first time." The place hasn't changed. We have.

This is a hopeful thought. We can revisit painful memories and find lessons in peace. We can revisit jealousy and find cooperation and trust. We can revisit fear and find that what we ran away from before was courage disguised. And Joy cannot be sought and found. It can only be found . . . at the place where we started.

Though we travel the world over to find the
beautiful, we must carry it with us or we find it
not.

—Ralph Waldo Emerson

Humor is not a joke or a trick. It is a presence in the universe which, like grace, shines on all of us.
                                            —Victor Borge

To benefit from the effects of humor you do not need to be able to tell jokes or funny stories. A sense of humor allows you to appreciate humor from a wide variety of sources.

A sense of humor can help you overlook the unattractive, tolerate the unpleasant, cope with the unexpected, and smile through the unbearable.
                                            —Moshe Waldoks

All truly great thoughts are conceived while walking.

—Friedrich Wilhelm Nietzsche

There are many physical benefits to walking: managing your weight, blood sugars, and stress levels; keeping your heart healthy; and increasing your energy and vitality. And there are less tangible benefits as well: enjoying the beauty around you, connecting with the beauty inside you, and experiencing great thoughts. Walks provide you a peaceful place to just be.

Laughter is a tranquilizer with no side effects.
—Anonymous

Not only that! When we laugh, the brain releases endorphins (the body's natural pain killer). If there is no pain, then the endorphins increase our sense of well-being—make us feel good. When life gets gloomy to the point where you don't feel like going to a funny movie or reading funny stories, look around. Children are a wonderful, nearly sure-fire source of laughter, exuberance, and joy. If there are no little people in your life right now, where can you do some volunteer work that would bring you in contact with some? Pets are another source of happy energy and funny situations. Take a walk to the park where there are sure to be children and dogs playing. (The exercise of the walk will raise your spirits, too.)

With fearful strains upon me, if I did not laugh, I would die.

—Abraham Lincoln

Both as a parent and as a president, Abraham Lincoln had enormous sorrows. His bright, inquiring mind and sense of humor helped bring him out of a dark depression and into the sunshine of laughter. We may not know Lincoln's resources for humor, but a much beloved resource in our time is the *I Love Lucy* show in re-runs. Ask people (at home, at work, at play) which are their favorites. Just talking about favorite Lucy episodes can (and usually does) bring laughter. Besides the candy factory episode, a favorite is the grape-stomping, wine-making of Lucy and Ethel. Their facial expressions are priceless.

We need to be careful about the difference between laughter which is healthy and creative and laughter which like Satan's is destructive—at someone else's expense . . . true laughter is freeing.
—Madeleine L'Engle

In her wonderful book, *Kitchen Table Wisdom*, Rachel Remen writes: "Life is the ultimate teacher, but it is usually through experience and not scientific research that we discover its deepest lessons." Science can measure the physical benefits of laughter, but the cleansing catharsis of a good belly laugh leaves us with no doubt.

The whole day stretches before us with unlimited opportunity! And what better way to appreciate that opportunity than by squandering it watching cartoons all day!

—Calvin to Hobbes

The Health Belief Model says that to take positive action for your health, you need three things: to understand the seriousness of your disease, to believe that you are personally vulnerable, and to have a strong, hopeful belief that you can do something to affect the outcome positively. To that let us add desire. Why do you want to live well? Your answer to "why" will motivate you to follow the "how." Friedrich Nietzsche said, "He who has a why to live can bear almost any how."

Can you make a list of all the whys you get out of bed in the morning?

I am—just as you are—a unique, never-to-be-repeated event in this universe, Therefore, I have— just as you have—a unique, never-to-be-repeated role in the world. Mine is a personal drama for which I am at once author, actor, and director.
—George A. Sheehan, MD

Novelist and poet Robert Louis Stevenson had tuberculosis all his life. Despite it, he lived adventurously and traveled widely. Of this challenge he said, "Life is not a matter of holding good cards. It's playing a poor hand well." That spirit of determination can guide each of us to live well with any challenge life brings.

Careful. We don't want to learn from this.
                    —Calvin and Hobbes

Consider your philosophy of life. How flexible is it? Does it help you to see events more as molehills than mountains? If your attitude toward life allows for ups and downs, you will be less stressed when they happen. A bumpy path is traveled more easily by someone who realizes that bumps are a part of life than it is by someone who demands that the road of life should always be smooth.

I myself am more and more inclined to agree with Omar and Satchel Paige as I grow older; Don't try to rewrite what the moving finger has writ, and don't ever look over your shoulder.

—Ogden Nash

Sometimes we just say, "That's life." Life is dynamic, ever-changing. Even the sources of stress change. Sometimes your family is a source of joy and sometimes a source of stress. Jobs are both fulfilling and frustrating. The same friend can provide both disappointment and delight. Even diabetes runs the gamut from teacher to tormenter. That's life.

How wonderful it is that nobody need wait a single moment before starting to improve the world.

—Anne Frank

Occasionally in life, it is good to be completely and totally humbled. I feel humble when I think on these words of the young woman who was eventually put to death in a Nazi concentration camp. And I start again to use compassion, forgiveness, and love as paths to improving life.

When anxious, uneasy and bad thoughts come, I go to the sea, and the sea drowns them out with its great wide sounds, cleanses me with its noise and imposes a rhythm upon everything in me that is bewildered and confused.

—Rainer Maria Rilke

The sea is not always available for us to find solace there. Nor is the beauty of the desert or the majesty of mountains an option when you live on the plains. Reflect a moment on how you could visit these other places when you cannot do so directly. Looking at a photograph on your desk? Listening to a recording of the natural sounds of that favorite place? Imaging yourself in the place you want to be? Getting together with friends who enjoy the same place? What works for you?

A journey of a thousand miles begins with a single step.

—Chinese proverb

What works for you to keep an exercise program going? Perhaps you don't like the word exercise, so you talk in terms of activity. That's fine. What keeps you active? Many of us today are finding that a pedometer or step-counter is a fun little motivator.

With a final goal of 10,000 steps a day, some people start at a lower goal, say 2,000 steps, and add 100 or 200 steps to their daily total at the beginning of each week, walking the new number of steps each day that week. They keep adding 100+ steps over weeks and months until they reach their goal of 10,000 steps a day. What an accomplishment!! And with so many benefits!

Often an extra loop around the neighborhood is all that's needed to complete your daily number of steps. Some people keep track of their miles and reward themselves when they reach certain mileposts.

*There is nothing—absolutely nothing—half so
much worth doing as simply messing about in boats.*
                                            —Kenneth Grahame

Someone told me that she finds a Zen garden to be very relaxing, freeing her, at least temporarily, from stress. I had never heard of a Zen garden, so she explained that it is a shallow box filled with sand. She uses a tiny rake to rake gently through the sand. As soon as she gracefully moved her hand in a raking gesture, I felt my knees go weak. My strong positive response comes from my love of boating. I have long associated sand with relaxation. That's an example of how the mind affects the body.

Let the past drift away with the water.
                                   —Japanese proverb

Rituals can help us by taking action. You might try listing your stresses on individual pieces of paper and burning them ceremoniously in a blazing fire in a fireplace or a bonfire on the beach. Throw a stick into a gutter that is carrying rain water toward the sewer and give the stick an identity, whether it is an experience from your past or a current source of stress. As purely symbolic as these activities are, they can be helpful because you are taking action.

In flood time you can see how some trees bend, and because they bend, even their twigs are safe, while stubborn trees are torn up roots and all.

—Sophocles

We can learn many lessons from nature. Saplings bend during storms and consequently do not break. We need to bend when life's storms hit us, so we won't break under the stress. I call that adaptability.

—from my book, *The Physician Within*

Be a willow with deep roots.

An idealist believes the short run doesn't count. A cynic believes the long run doesn't matter. A realist believes that what is done or left undone in the short run determines the long run.

—Sydney J. Harris

This brings us to the old debate about managing blood sugars closely. Some said that it did not matter if blood glucose (blood sugar) were closely managed or not. They believed people simply got complications no matter what. Those who felt the long run doesn't matter had a "live for today" approach to life with no regard for the future. The results of the Diabetes Control and Complications Trial (DCCT) of people with type 1 diabetes and the United Kingdom Prospective Diabetes Study (UKPDS) of people with type 2 diabetes support the belief of the realist. Managing your blood sugars today means you will have fewer or no complications tomorrow. Do you have a list of all the reasons you want to be healthy today and for many years to come?

The rain to the wind said,
"You push and I'll pelt."
They so smote the garden bed
That the flowers actually knelt,
And lay lodged—though not dead.
I know how the flowers felt.

—Robert Frost

Have you ever felt like those flowers? Most of us have. What were the circumstances that brought you to your knees? What brought you back?

Twenty years from now you will be more disappointed by the things you didn't do than by the ones you did do. So throw off the bowlines. Sail away from the safe harbor. Catch the trade winds in your sails. Explore. Dream. Discover.

—Mark Twain

There still are people who think that diabetes limits them in what they can do (travel? running in a marathon?) and experience (having a child? going to medical school?). What dreams do you have for your life? Will your health care provider support you in getting there? Do not accept any limitation that you absolutely do not have to accept—especially if the limitation is fear or pride.

Hope is the thing with feathers that perches in the soul and sings the tune without the words and never stops at all. And, sweetest in the gale is heard.
—Emily Dickinson

Life's darkest, most difficult moments help us to discover and appreciate this wonderful, never-ending source of strength and comfort: Hope. Much has been written about hope, but it will be your own direct, personal experience that will be the most valuable way for you to connect to it and receive its power. Have you had such an experience? Choice plays a big role here.

Worry never robs tomorrow of its sorrow, it only saps today of its joy.

—Leo Buscaglia

Whether you are a person who has diabetes, or the parent or grandparent of a child with diabetes, the spouse of someone with diabetes, or a friend, you probably get concerned about diabetes. Concern comes out of the awareness that diabetes is serious. However, when concern turns into worry, it can become unhealthy. Worry can create more problems for your loved one as well as for you and the rest of the family and friends. Talk with a member of the health care team to express and deal with issues of concern. Do all you can, then let go. Don't waste your energy on worry.

Let me tell you the secret that has led me to my goal: my strength lies solely in my tenacity.

—Louis Pasteur

Do you enjoy reading famous people's secrets of success? What makes these secrets so valuable is that they apply to our own lives, too. Living well with diabetes is supported by many personal qualities. To determination, desire, and sense of humor, we need to add tenacity. What helps a scientist keep going no matter how many failures he has experienced is a character trait that leads to success in living with diabetes—tenacity.

*If I had but three loaves of bread, I would sell one
and buy hyacinths, for they would feed my soul.*
                                                 —the Koran

What nourishment do you feed your soul? Here
are some suggestions to help you make your own list of
soul food: philosophy, poetry, literature, religious or
spiritual teachings, nature, art, and altruism (giving
help to others). We need regular spiritual nourishment. We all encounter times of questioning, times of
feeling fragile or vulnerable, momentary anger and
sadness over disease or disability. There are simply
some days when we are "down." That's the time for
soul food! With regular spiritual nourishment, we have
a reserve to call on whenever necessary.

The best most of us can do is to be a Poet an hour a day. Take the hour when we run or play tennis or golf or garden; take that hour away from being serious adults and become serious beginners.
                                    —George A. Sheehan, MD

A friend who is a cardiologist recommends exercise (activity) to his patients not only for the physical benefit, but also for the spiritual benefit. He believes that one of the most important benefits of exercise is that it increases our self-esteem. In lectures he uses a slide showing a woman running up a hill. She is all alone. On the picture are the words: The Sound of Cheering from Within. The message is that we do this activity for our own health and well-being. We are not doing it to please our health care team, boss, spouse, children, or friends. The benefit—and the pride—is ours.

There is nothing like returning to a place that remains unchanged to find the ways in which you yourself have altered.

—Nelson Mandela

Once you are diagnosed with diabetes, every part of your life is like this return trip. There, nothing has changed, but it seems that everything has changed for you. With the help of your health care team, you will find ways to engage in life as you knew it and enjoyed it before you were diagnosed. Be sure to let them know what aspects of your new lifestyle are troubling or difficult. Diabetes educators use their heads as well as their hearts to support you in your ongoing quest for a fulfilling life.

*You can do what you have to do, and sometimes
you can do it even better than you think you can.*
—Jimmy Carter

In the 1950s, the diabetic meal plan included 5, 10, 15, and 20% fruits (based on sugar content). Most food was weighed on a gram scale. Heavy glass syringes with big steel needles were the only way to deliver insulin. Urine was tested for sugar by putting 5 drops of urine and 10 drops of water into a test tube and adding a chemical tablet that caused the mixture to boil, transforming it to a color that was then compared with a color chart reading from negative to positive 4. Parents of infants with diabetes had to "test" a wet diaper. Without blood glucose monitoring, people had to rely on symptoms of low blood sugar to alert them of the need for food to prevent serious hypoglycemia. People did what they needed to do.

Think about when you were diagnosed. What were the issues that seemed to be huge stumbling blocks then? Did you handle them? Did you do even better than you thought you could?

A little of what you fancy does you good.
                                        —Marie Lloyd

Dietary recommendations seem to change constantly. We've seen surprising swings in advice, from "Don't eat sugar at all" to "You can work sweets into your meal plan." There is wisdom in indulging a little bit in what you want, so that you don't feel deprived. Feelings of deprivation often lead to overindulgence. The key is in the phrase "working sweets in." Doing this sensibly means that you still follow a nutritious meal plan, but you include a *little* of what you fancy, so that you feel satisfied.

A *lot* of what you fancy can be harmful.

Choose well; your choice is brief, and yet endless.
—Goethe

This thought has profound significance for moral and ethical choices. But we can also apply it to our own diabetes care, where the daily choices we make can have long-lasting repercussions. An even more practical application can be found in this light-hearted, familiar saying:

A moment at the lips . . . forever on the hips.

Mistakes are, after all, the foundations of truth, and if a [person] does not know what a thing is, it is at least an increase in knowledge if he knows what it is not.

—Carl Jung

Diabetes management is an imprecise science. We make mistakes all the time, but we learn all the time too. Predicting the impact of a particular food on blood glucose levels is tricky, and sometimes the first indication is your blood glucose reading after a meal. Embrace the wisdom of Jung's thought, but instead of using the word "mistake," think of it as "experiment." People with diabetes are their own personal scientists. Through experimentation you learn, daily, what works and what does not work.

The trail is the thing, not the end of the trail. Travel too fast and you miss all you are traveling for.
—Louis L'Amour

The pace of our lives often seems to be set at fast forward—causing us to miss not only the beauty around us, but also the point of life. Stop in the middle of your day and do a replay of where you've been, what you've seen, and what you've done. What beauty did you encounter along the way? Are you enjoying the journey?

In solitude we give passionate attention to our lives,
to our memories, to the details around us.

—Virginia Woolf

In solitude we allow the dust of life to settle. We evaluate where we've been and where we want to go. Without the distractions of today's fast-paced life, we can make important choices about how to live. Look at your calendar. Carve out some time. Make a date with yourself . . . alone.

Behavior is a function of meaning.
—Robert Anderson

We tell ourselves that a sweet sandwich-type cookie is simply a wonderful treat, and our mouths might even water at the thought. Now, try a new thought: The filling of a sandwich cookie is solid shortening sweetened with sugar. Picture a can of solid shortening. Would you want to eat a spoonful? If a sack of sugar were placed in front of you, would you really be tempted to eat it?

Cookies like these are solid shortening sweetened with sugar. They contribute to weight gain and to increases in cholesterol and blood glucose levels. Could this new definition, this new meaning, lead you to change your behavior?

There is nothing to it. You only have to hit the right notes at the right time and the instrument plays itself.

—Johann Sebastian Bach

Similarly, there's nothing to managing diabetes. Just make sure that the food you eat, the activities you engage in, and the medications you take are all timed right and perfectly balanced, and diabetes just manages itself! Each day, we engage in the art of living well, and when we succeed, we are every bit as much of a master artist as Bach or Rembrandt.

Diabetes is not the leading cause of blindness.
Unmanaged diabetes is.
　　　　　　　　　—William Howard Polonsky

What a healthy and hopeful perspective this is! We are too often surrounded by negative thoughts and dire predictions. Hopelessness fed by negative beliefs can lead to self-fulfilling prophecies. Hope*ful*ness fed by positive beliefs can also lead to self-fulfilling prophecies. We need to choose our thoughts carefully. They determine our direction as well as our destination.

JUNE 16

To map out a course of action and follow it to an end requires some of the same courage that a soldier needs.

—Ralph Waldo Emerson

Life with diabetes, or any chronic disease, can be viewed as a battle. If this is a metaphor that works for you, then map out your course of action. Take a few minutes to list the dangers of the battlefield and then write down your plan of action for avoiding those dangers.

Diabetes research has concluded that well-managed diabetes can help you to avoid the complications of blindness, kidney failure, and nerve damage. Your health care team can recommend a course of action for managing your blood sugars closely. But it is you who must find the courage to follow it "to an end." Use inspiring thoughts such as the ones throughout this book to stoke the embers of courage within you.

Success is to be measured not so much by the position that one has reached in life as by the obstacles which he has overcome.

—Booker T. Washington

I watched a marathon in which I knew one of the runners. She has diabetes and wears an insulin pump. Partway through the 26-mile run, her infusion set fell off—the sweat loosened the adhesive. She had to stop and insert a new infusion set. She stopped several more times to monitor her blood glucose, eat, or take insulin. Yet she finished the marathon. Her time may not have been a winning one, but she was a winner.

Pilots and ships' captains must frequently check their bearings to keep on course, just as people with diabetes frequently monitor their blood glucose to see what adjustments they need to make. Just as a ship's captain stays on course because she has learned how to adjust the sails, people with diabetes learn how to adjust food, activity, and medication to stay on course.

The dog was created for children. He is the god of frolic.

—Henry Ward Beecher

Pets are for the child who resides in each of us—whether we are child or adult. A nurse in a stress-management seminar once said, "When I come home from work feeling really tired, I see my two dogs in the window, all excited to see me, and I forget that I'm tired and I feel renewed energy to play with them." And the play (or frolic) turns into more renewal! It is no wonder that research has shown that owning a cat or dog can lower blood pressure and make stress more manageable.

Outside of a dog, books are a man's best friend. Inside of a dog, it's too dark to read.

—Groucho Marx

Example is the school of mankind, and they will learn at no other.

—Edmund Burke

From whose example have you learned? What examples have you followed in your lifestyle choices? What are some actions you have taken in regards to eating, exercise, and stress management that you learned, not from a class, lecture, or book, but from someone's example?

If you are not satisfied or happy with any of these actions, seek other examples to follow. You will find what you seek.

*Each of us must work for his own improvement,
and at the same time share a general responsibility
for all humanity.*

—Marie Curie

Marie Curie's wisdom builds on that of Edmund Burke. Just as each of us learns from the examples around us, so do we teach by the example we set. Who are *you* teaching? *What* are you teaching?

We all have big changes in our lives that are more or less a second chance.

—Harrison Ford

People often report that their diagnosis of diabetes was just that: a second chance. It gave them the opportunity to focus on how they want to live their lives, to start making healthy choices, and to define or redefine their life's goal to live well. How has your life changed since you were diagnosed? Have you taken advantage of the opportunity you've been given for a second chance?

It's the movies that have really been running things in America ever since they were invented. They show you what to do, how to do it, when to do it, how to feel about it, and how to look how you feel about it.

—Andy Warhol

Whether you agree or disagree with this opinion, it can generate an enlightening discussion. Do you remember when there was a lot of cigarette smoking in movies? It was the sophisticated, "beautiful" people who ceremoniously lit up and dramatically blew the smoke out. Do you think these scenes affected the behavior of viewers? What other behaviors or attitudes do you think have been influenced by movies? Can movies also affect the way we see ourselves?

*The lesson in running brooks is that motion is a
great purifier and health producer. When the brook
ceases to run, it soon stagnates. In motion it soon
leaves all mud and sediment behind.*

—John Burroughs
The Gospel of Nature

A woman with arthritis told how she kept her joints from getting too stiff. She chose to work the front desk of her sister's hotel, where she had to keep getting up to register new guests when they arrived. There are lessons to be learned from nature, which includes all the brave men, women, and children we encounter daily. Recognize that each person has a story. Listen to their stories. What lessons can they teach you?

If you let cloudy water settle, it will become clear.
If you let your upset mind settle, your course will
also become clear.

—Buddhist saying

How do you settle your mind when you are upset? You could leave the room; take a walk; drink some cold water; meditate or pray; get a good night's sleep; talk with a calming, trusted friend; focus on peaceful thoughts; or simply distract yourself, so you don't think about the situation that has made you upset. Sometimes by *not* thinking about a situation, the course becomes clear.

I used to play Mozart when I was stressed. There were so many little black notes to concentrate on that I could not possibly continue to dwell on whatever was stressful.

The best thing about the future is that it comes only one day at a time.

—Abraham Lincoln

Periodically, we need to be reminded to live this moment only. By focusing on the here and now, rather than dwelling on the past or future, we are less likely to be overwhelmed. Numerous writers have expressed this thought, perhaps no one more beautifully than C. S. Lewis in *Letter to an American Lady*.

We must try to take life moment by moment. The actual present is usually pretty tolerable, I think, if only we refrain from adding to its burden that of the past and the future.

Nine-tenths of wisdom is being wise in time.
—Theodore Roosevelt

People sometimes put off self-care, thinking they'll start practicing a more healthy lifestyle when they retire, or when they have more time, or at the first sign of a serious problem. But sometimes that time never comes, and the first heart attack is not a wake-up call, it's the end. Are you living wisely? If not, when are you going to start?

Tomorrow is often the busiest day of the week.
—Spanish proverb

Who has not sat tense before his own heart's curtain?

—Rainer Maria Rilke

The experience of being diagnosed with a serious illness is not the only time people might be connected to thoughts of the final curtain—their death. Such thoughts can reappear throughout our lives and can cause stress and tension, a sort of "dis-ease" of our emotions and spirit. One of the best ways to cope with the stress caused by these thoughts is to reframe it, or change our way of thinking about it. An example of reframing is changing the thought "I'm doomed to go blind" to "Because I have the knowledge, skills, tools, and support to manage my diabetes, I can do much to prevent blindness and live a full and happy life."

I thought my life would be more interesting with a musical score and a laugh track.

—Calvin and Hobbes

Change your thoughts and you change your world.
—Norman Vincent Peale

Speaking of change: Here is a fun perspective from the queen of humor, Barbara Johnson: "Laughter is like changing a baby's diaper. It doesn't permanently solve any problem, but it does make things more acceptable for a while."

Naps are nature's way of reminding you that life is nice—like a beautiful, softly swinging hammock strung between birth and infinity.

—Peggy Noonan

Take some time for daydreaming. Whether you stretch out on a hammock, sit in a comfortable chair, wiggle your toes in the sand, or stare into the dancing flames in a fireplace, find the setting that encourages daydreaming. Reconnect with all that makes life nice by taking trips down Memory Lane and Wishful Road. And when you cannot be in the setting of your choice, visualize yourself there. We all need to take mini-vacations away from the day-to-day stresses of life.

Inside myself is a place where I live all alone and that's where I renew my springs that never dry up.
—Pearl S. Buck

Reflection is similar to daydreaming. The one difference may be that in daydreaming we go outside of ourselves and in reflection we go inside to visit the springs of wisdom within us. Renewal comes from the nourishment of great thoughts, beautiful sights, and inspiring sounds. What do you do when you're feeling parched? Where do you go to renew yourself?

Your success and happiness lie in you . . . Resolve to keep happy, and your joy and you shall form an invincible host against difficulties.

—Helen Keller

Summer's overall theme is joy. Our willingness to engage in diabetes self-management is fueled by our desire to enjoy life. A Kanem proverb from a twelfth century African civilization invites you to consider your own philosophy and reason for managing diabetes: "We will water the thorn for the sake of the rose."

We can reflect on the life cycle of flowers, ponder the metaphor of oak trees, and play with the thought that even a blade of grass has its own angel. Emerson said that "the earth laughs in flowers." Such thoughts can awaken you to the beauty and joy that surround you everyday—whether you're in a garden or a grocery store.

Summer also brings the power outages of summer storms and chores like mowing the lawn. Make some metaphors: Power outages are low blood sugars that can be prevented or treated. Mowing a lawn symbolizes the routine of life. I have to mow the lawn. I have to brush my teeth. I have to monitor blood glucose. I have to do some chores in life. I get to fly kites, hike, go on picnics, pick flowers, play—and experience creativity and joy.

What do we live for if not to make the world less difficult for each other?

—George Eliot

What is currently weighing you down? With pen and paper handy, empty your head and your heart of all that concerns you at present. Write it down. Then, focus your attention on the spiritual wind that lifts your soul.

"Spiritual wind" can be a metaphor for the forces of light, joy, rejuvenation, faith, and hope. Now, take up your pen and fill your paper and your heart with everything you can think of that lifts your soul.

According to Dr. Rachel Naomi Remen, author of *Kitchen Table Wisdom*, the purpose of life is to grow in wisdom and to learn how to love better. She believes this can be accomplished through service to others.

Consider the ways you can be of service to those around you. For example, the simple act of holding the door for another person is a service. Have your experiences of service uplifted you? List some of the possibilities for service today.

And this our life . . . Finds tongues in trees, books in running brooks, Sermons in stones, and good in everything.

—William Shakespeare

We used to have two huge, silver maple trees in our yard. After a particularly cold winter, one of them died. I was really stunned. The tree had seemed so healthy . . . and it had been part of our yard, almost like a member of our family.

We asked a tree specialist about the situation, and he said that silver maples have roots close to the surface. So, when there is a bitterly cold winter, the roots are affected by the cold. We decided to make a large ring around the remaining silver maple. The ring is bounded by large, round rocks and is filled with wood shavings, a blanket of insulation to protect the roots.

Nature had reinforced yet another important life lesson: Prevention. This lesson caused me to ask myself, "Am I doing as much for my own current and future health as I am for our tree?" I can meditate on that thought after a vigorous walk followed by a cool-down in the backyard. And, while cooling down, I look for lessons elsewhere.

No pessimist ever discovered the secrets of the stars
or sailed to an uncharted land or opened a new
heaven to the human spirit.

—Helen Keller

Optimism is mostly a cherished attribute. People understand that life is better when they can view it with hope rather than despair. Dr. Robert Schuller refers to optimism as "possibility thinking." From sociologists to historians to motivational speakers, we hear about the "can do" approach to life.

Optimism has built civilizations, negotiated unlikely peace treaties, started businesses, and discovered cures. In day-to-day living, it is optimism that means diabetes and joy can exist side by side in life . . . in each life affected by diabetes.

Some people seem to be naturally optimistic, but all of us have pessimism and cynicism knocking on the door . . . daily. The choice for all of us is to decide who we will let in the door—the door to our minds. Reflect on the thoughts that nourish your mind on a daily basis. Choose your mental nourishment as carefully as you choose physical nourishment.

It's okay to have butterflies in your stomach. Just get them to fly in formation.

—Helen Keller

A friend of mine shared a delightful way in which she helps herself regain a sense of control when her life is out of balance, stressed, or simply too busy. She walks into the family room of their home and looks at the shelf holding her collection of ducks. She reports: "I feel reassured and calm when I see that *somewhere* in my life . . . I have all my ducks in a row!"

Barbara Johnson carried a variation of that theme in her newsletter *The Love Line*: "When Life seems chaotic and you feel overwhelmed, take a deep breath, get your ducks in a row . . . and take 'em in the tub with you!"

Humor, a brief break, a new perspective. . . . You don't need a collection of ducks to tap into those stress managers. Consider how you use humor and a break to give yourself a new perspective.

. . . to know even one life has breathed easier because you lived. This is to have succeeded.
　　　　　　　　　—Ralph Waldo Emerson

Support is the reason that strong people are strong. We all need to feel supported. Years ago, former President Gerald Ford's son Steven spoke to 400 women in Minneapolis on "Life in the White House." He told us funny stories, especially about his teenage perspective on having to include a secret service agent in all of his activities!

Suddenly he stopped and said, "Before I forget, I want to say, 'Thank you'." His mother, Betty Ford, had had a mastectomy when he was a teenager. He knew it had been a difficult experience for her, and he asked her how she'd made it.

She said it was the cards, notes, and letters from women all over the United States who wrote to tell her they had had the same surgery. They made it, and she was in their prayers.

Believing that at least one woman in the group may have written to his mother, he thanked us all. So, who needs support? The first lady of the United States of America . . . and each and every one of us.

After enlightenment, there's still the laundry.
                                    —Chinese proverb

Being "in the moment" is not mysterious. Being in the moment is being aware of life, of what is happening right now, and not thinking about last week or tomorrow. This is the only way to receive the messages of the moment. There are practical benefits to this practice as well as the celebrated rewards of peace and appreciation of beauty. For example, we can see the impact of food and exercise on blood glucose levels right now.

Being in the moment also means that we notice the tiny buds on the trees in Spring and then, the fullness of the leaves when Summer takes over Spring's task. Being in the moment as we talk with a friend or help a stranger helps us see love in action.

Being in the moment helps me keep my balance. I need to think beautiful thoughts to feed my soul, to encounter great wisdom to enlighten my mind, and to experience blood glucose results to guide my decisions. Life is lived in both the huge and small, the eloquent and the humble, the grand Aha's and the simple, necessary tasks.

I was studying Shakespeare in Europe in 1968 when Robert Kennedy and Martin Luther King, Jr., were assassinated. My sadness and shock were great, but I couldn't find language to express my feelings. Then I read *Measure for Measure* by William Shakespeare, and the following lines flew directly to my heart.

But man, proud man, dressed in a little brief authority plays such fantastic tricks before high heaven as makes the angels weep.

The image of angels weeping with me gave a context to my experience: A loss of such magnitude that the angels wept. This idea of a divine support group gave me strength and started my healing. I felt better because I had connected with words that gave meaning to my deep feelings. And I felt lifted up by angelic images more powerful than words.

Healing is necessary before we can find the energy to manage diabetes and all the other life tasks before us. Be open to the many and, often unexpected, sources for healing.

Go with the flow.

—Popular saying

If Life is the university, then Nature is surely one of its noblest, most honored professors. The Mississippi River is nicknamed, the "Mighty Mississippi" for good reason. Strong current etches shorelines like an artist's paintbrush creates a picture. One day as I was enjoying the ever-changing view of the river's shoreline from a boat, I saw another aspect of the current. Although the boat's engines had been cut back, the boat was moving swiftly downstream.

Swift current increases fuel efficiency when one is going downstream. Likewise, the strong current makes an upstream trip more difficult, and much more fuel is consumed in the process.

Professor Nature raised its eyebrows in lovely, puffy, white clouds. The question posed to me was: As current is to the river, what are the outside forces in your life that help you get where you're going more efficiently, with less drain on your energy? What are the outside forces that make "headway" in diabetes or any life task more difficult?

If you hold on to the handle, she said, it's easier to maintain the illusion of control. But it's more fun if you just let the wind carry you.

—Brian Andreas

A professor of Classics wrote that the word "yes" is the most powerful word in the English language. I am reminded of a time Robert Fulghum came to Minneapolis. Fulghum, a popular author, made it known that he had a fantasy of conducting an orchestra. The marketing director of the Minneapolis Chamber Symphony wrote and offered her orchestra.

He accepted the invitation, but shortly after, he learned of serious political and financial difficulties within the Chamber Symphony. As he flew to Minneapolis, he wondered if any musicians would be there. When he arrived, the stage was full of musicians. Fulghum said, "The fact that there are musicians on stage means the 'Yes!' goes on."

When have you been carried by the Yes or have you chosen Yes? Consider a situation you are facing today. What does it mean to choose Yes?

Earth laughs in flowers.

—Ralph Waldo Emerson

Smile whenever you see flowers erupting from the ground. What is it that caused the earth to laugh there?

Were the daffodils a response to a gentle tickling created by a rake?

Did the tulips emerge when rain trickled down and the earth chuckled in delight?

Is the earth's floral laughter its way to express joy and gratitude to its creator?

I want to think so. I am inspired by this thought. I wonder how I am expressing my joy and gratitude?

A faithful friend is the medicine of life.
                                    —Ecclesiastes 6:16

The notion that an apple a day keeps us healthy is supported by research, but so is the power and importance of social support: we need friends.

Giving friendship may be even more health-promoting than being on the receiving end of friendship. Dr. Hans Selye, a Montreal physician who was considered an expert in stress management, reported that giving of himself to help others was the single greatest stress reducer in his life.

To receive the "medicine" of friendship, give friendship. As is said about love, the more you give, the more you receive.

Today's mighty oak is just yesterday's nut that held its ground.

—Author unknown

Some of the scariest storms I have experienced have been in the summer . . . especially the storms at night. The crashing thunder and awesome lightning make me feel small and insignificant. Strong wind is especially frightening at night because I can't see what it's doing.

I remember having to go out one night in such a storm to check on the rainspouts. A gust of wind nearly knocked me over. I found my way to our oak tree and grabbed hold. As I regained my balance, I felt a surge of comfort and security, a gift from the large, solid oak tree.

We all encounter storms in our lives. Diabetes can be one of them. Each of us needs to find our tree. Hold on. Receive its support. Its many branches can include family, friends, church and synagogue, the heroes and heroines of life past and present.

At a party one evening, I overheard my husband telling someone: "The best thing that ever happened to me was marrying someone with diabetes. We live such a healthy life."

He is my oak. Reflect on yours.

*Good and evil, reward and punishment are the only
motives to a rational creature: these are the spurs
and reins whereby all mankind are set on work,
and guided.*

—John Locke

If rewards were not important, I doubt there
would be trophies for athletic achievement, gold stars
on papers, or corporate awards for departments and
individuals.

Rewards can be things, like trophies or medals.
Rewards can be feelings of self-confidence as we celebrate a job well done. Most of us look forward to some
reward for our efforts.

In the 1970s during lectures, I made the observation that there was an odd sort of reward system in
diabetes management. It seemed to be: "If you take
really good care of yourself, maybe in 15 or 20 years
you won't go blind." Negative, half-promises far out
in the future are poor rewards for today's behavior.

You need a short-term reward, if not right away,
then soon. A reward gives us a boost to keep working
on behaviors like regular exercise, blood glucose monitoring, and healthful eating. Rewards are important.
What rewards do you respond to most positively?

When you listen with your soul, you come into
rhythm and unity with the music of the universe.
　　　　　　　　　　　　　　　—John O'Donohue

Sometimes I need inspiration from great, thunderous, amazing, and magnificent music. Whether orchestral or vocal, the music floods me with its power and lifts me above the world that causes distress.

Sometimes I need quiet inspiration, the kind that comes as I sit on a dock at sunset watching a distant city skyscape or the forest's tree-lined contour.

And then, I am amazed by the silence . . . the quiet around me allowing the music within me to be heard.

A merry heart doeth good like a medicine.
—Proverbs 17:22

If King Solomon had written a book on the effects of humor on health, he might have called it "Amusing Grace." Surely, it is humor that warms us and strengthens us. Some people feel in control over anything they can laugh at or about. The following story is an example of being in control of an otherwise difficult situation.

A woman who'd had both legs amputated below the knee left her prostheses in a changing room at the club when she exercised in the swimming pool. Because the door left eighteen inches or so open to the floor, people could see two legs, and some wondered if a woman in the changing room were in need of help. To deal with the curious and the concerned, she put a sign on the door: "My legs are resting. I'm in the pool."

Joy is not in things; it is in us.

—Richard Wagner

Famous people often get asked for advice, formulas for success, or descriptions of their personal happiness. The English poet, John Keats, offered this:

Give me books, fruit, French wine, fine weather,
and a little music out of doors, played by someone
I do not know.

If you suddenly found yourself famous, how would you respond to a journalist who asked you the question: "What is it in life that makes you happy?"

Then, how would you respond to the question: "What is your source of joy?"

JULY 18

The truth is rarely pure and never simple.
—Oscar Wilde

Comedian David Letterman remarked once that he was struck by the wording on a bag he saw in a hardware store: "Worm and Grub Killer." Letterman said that if we named products based on outcomes, then "candy bars" really should be called "fat-boy zit bars." Whereas a "juicy steak" may sound appealing, "blubber" and "lard" usually don't.

Finish the following descriptions à la Letterman:

rich desserts would be _____

high-fat meats would be _____

high-salt, high-fat snacks would be _____

fast food would be _____

After smiling about our creative responses, we might even feel like making healthier choices.

The average child laughs 146 times a day. The
average adult laughs 4 times a day.

—Anonymous

When blood sugar gets low, quite commonly a person's disposition sours. One day when my son was about seven years old, he noticed that I was "out of sorts." He looked at me intently and said: "Are ya low, Mom?" His innocent question startled me into perspective. I said to him: "No, I'm not low, I was just being crabby . . . and I'm sorry."

That experience became a source of humor for our family as we gave exaggerated versions of the question: "Are ya low, Mom?" The story became a way to balance as we all came to realize the value of chilling out when any of us was under stress. We learned to respect one another's space and individual needs for regaining perspective.

When an occasionally grumpy little boy got off the school bus, I gave him time and space.

Everyone needs that, not just people with diabetes.

Some people regard discipline as a chore. For me, it is a kind of order that sets me free to fly.
—Julie Andrews

There have to be times when the disciplined life of diabetes self-management seems like a chore. But, can it also be a structure that allows for greater freedom?

With the discipline of a well-planned series of meals, extra food, and blood glucose monitoring materials, people can take diabetes on canoe trips, climbing expeditions, vacations, and all the day-to-day activities that include work as well as play.

Diabetes can even accompany us on spontaneous excursions. Prior planning sets the stage for spontaneity. Extra food in the glove box of the car, a book bag, briefcase, or purse can supply the fuel for a flight of fantasy. If your blood glucose meter is a daily companion, a safe landing is likely to result.

Set yourself free to fly.

Every blade of grass has its Angel that bends over it and whispers, "Grow, grow."

—The Talmud

Some people see angels as winged, ethereal creatures playing golden harps. Others think of angels as being invisible but with a very real presence in their lives. Still others give angelic qualities to the people in their lives who seem to "be there" whenever help is needed with a pot of soup, a shoveled walk, or a cheery phone call. In all cases, angels are the forces of good.

Reflect on the "angels"—visible and invisible—in your life that have encouraged your growth and healing. Have there been times when you were someone's angel?

The intelligent want self-control; children want candy.

—Rumi

Meditating about angels in our lives can bring some questions to the surface. Do we always recognize angels?

Is it possible that people who annoy us are actually angels? Some of the annoyance that many of us experience with people in relation to our diabetes, is that they "nag" us. "Are you testing?" asks a parent. "Should you be eating that?" asks a spouse, coworker, or friend. "How's the weight?" asks a health care professional.

It's time to ask ourselves: "Are they nagging me or are they genuinely concerned and just asking me how I'm doing?"

Is it possible that their questions are motivated by their love and their desire to see us do well and be well? To grow, grow.

Maybe they don't fully recognize who we are. Are you a rebel? Or are you a responsible person making the best choices you can?

Maybe we all need to talk more.

Be still and know that I am God.

—Psalm 46:10

Mary Casey, chaplain at Fairview University Medical Center in Minneapolis, combines breathing and mental imagery in meditations with patients. She says that when we focus on our breathing, we let go of distracting thoughts. To open to healing messages, it helps to focus on a peaceful place, such as a setting by a lake or river.

Mary invites people to imagine the waves of the lake taking anxiety from the center of the lake to the shore where God's arms receive it. The wave is then sent back out cleansed. God's arms are much like the shore of the lake, able to receive and hold anything brought to them. Mary refers to this image as a "place of grace," and as we "lean into it," we can hear God's gentle voice saying the beautiful words:

> Be still and know that I am God
> Be still and know that I am
> Be still and know that I
> Be still and know that
> Be still and know
> Be still and
> Be still
> Be

Oh that I had wings like a dove! I would fly away and be at rest; yea, I would wander afar, I would lodge in the wilderness.

—Psalm 55:6–7

My friend Mary used to plant daffodils in the woods behind her house . . . not in a row, but at random. Always, it was a delightful surprise to spot them. She called me one day and said simply, "What a wonderful day to be a daffodil."

My imagination did the rest. I pictured myself as a daffodil gently bobbing in the breeze. Stress was gone. I smiled all day whenever I thought about being a daffodil protected by the surrounding woods, gently kissed by streaks of sunlight, and tickled by gentle winds. Although we don't have wings to carry us, we do have imagination.

*Look for the rainbow, that gracious thing, made up
of tears and light.*
> —Samuel Taylor Coleridge

We see rainbows when there has been rain. It is a natural phenomenon caused by the combination of rain and sunshine. The rainbow was God's promise to Noah and future generations that never again would the entire earth be covered with water. The flood that covered the whole earth and caused Noah to build the ark and save pairs of animals would not recur.

But, God did not promise an end to rain. Indeed, the earth cannot survive if we do not receive rain on a regular and restorative basis. So it is with our lives.

No one can promise us an end to our tears. But the rainbow reminds us that life will not be only tears. We will experience light—as laughter, as love, as joy, as renewed hope. The rainbow also reminds us that we cannot have only light. We need both sunshine and rain, joy and tears . . . for it is their combination that produces beauty and beams a promise.

The rainbow's beauty is today's pleasure and tomorrow's promise that there is always hope.

The river is a wonderful book with a new story to tell everyday.

—Mark Twain

Life provides many classrooms—from libraries and schools to rivers and mountains. The river is my favorite classroom.

Whether the river takes us to towns, festivals, or fishing, there are stories to hear at every bend. But, when we are very still and watch the river and listen carefully, we hear our own stories . . . welling up from the river within us.

The river has taught me to listen; you will learn from it, too. The river knows everything; one can learn everything from it.

—Hermann Hesse

We will water the thorn for the sake of the rose.
—Kanem proverb

Prevention is a very important part of diabetes self-care. We want to prevent the complications of diabetes. But prevention is not the whole picture. Can you imagine getting out of bed in the morning, stretching, and saying: "Well, another day to prevent blindness"?

Beyond prevention of early death, disability, and disease, there is the promotion of life, health, and well-being. The reason we eat nutritiously, take medication (if prescribed), exercise, and monitor blood glucose is so that we can enjoy life.

I love the image of the hearth as a place of home, a place of warmth and return. In everyone's inner solitude there is that bright and warm hearth.
—John O'Donohue

Zig Ziglar, a motivational expert, compares motivation to a fire in a fireplace. When the fire ceases to burn, you take a poker, poke the logs a few times, and soon have a roaring blaze again. In poking the logs, the movement of air creates a partial vacuum in the fireplace. Since nature abhors a vacuum, fresh air rushes in to fill the space, bringing the additional oxygen that ignites the smoldering logs and . . . you have a fire!

According to Ziglar's analogy, people are like those logs. Internally there is a smoldering fire, and often all we need is a little stoking from some outside force to get our fire going again.

We need "pokers" to rekindle our inner fire.

Who, what, where are the pokers in your life?

Singin' in the rain, just singin' in the rain.
What a glorious feeling, I'm happy again.
—Arthur Freed

A sign at a summer camp said: GREAT WALK. I had been told that the path was indeed a great walk, both for the natural wonders of plants, flowers, trees, ponds, and resident animals, as well as for the rigor of the physical workout. I reflected on the sign and thought of its deeper meaning in my life's walk.

Just as rain gear helps me enjoy the sight of a raindrop splashing off a glistening leaf, so does the "rain gear" of blood glucose meter and carbohydrates help me engage more fully in life.

If Life is to be a great walk, then our knapsack must be packed with all that we will need physically, mentally, and spiritually: granola bars to feed your body, books to fuel your mind, and experiences that your soul uses to nourish your heart.

Your body reveals you within and without. It tells the perceptive observer your philosophy, your view of the universe.

—George A. Sheehan, MD

The state of Victoria in Australia is greatly committed to promoting health. Car races are sponsored by Vic Health Promotion. Cigarettes are heavily taxed, and the taxes support health promotion.

The billboards are wonderful. They advertise exercise and lifelong, healthy activity. They show active children, adolescents, young adults, adults, and seniors. The message is one of health and self. Health cannot just "happen." Health is a direct result of choices we make.

What billboards do you see in your neighborhood, on your way to work, or driving other places? What are they promoting? What is the message? Most importantly, what are the "billboards" in your mind? What are the messages you choose (or allow) on display in your mind?

The blessings for which we hunger are not to be found in other places or people. These gifts can only be given to you by yourself.

—John O'Donohue

Good quality of life is what each of us seeks. The definition of quality depends on individual goals, needs, and values. Reflect on what quality of life means to you. This is the foundation of your motivation, the reason that you are willing to manage diabetes day to day, hour by hour.

People report the following definitions of quality of life:

- feeling well so that I can enjoy family life
- being able to participate in all areas of my life with energy
- being free of complications of diabetes
- living fully in spite of complications
- having physical and mental energy and spiritual peace

Over the next several pages, we consider a process that is a way to achieve a better quality of life. Ask yourself **questions.** If life is a journey, then it is a **question** that begins it and questions that make us continue the journey.

Shall we make a new rule of life from tonight:
always try to be a little kinder than is necessary?
— Sir James M. Barrie

Uplift yourself and others. This energizes you spiritually. Thirty years ago, I met a woman from rural Minnesota. She knew I had diabetes. She said one sentence to me: "I just want you to know that I have had diabetes for 44 years."

I drank her in! She looked perfectly healthy. At that point I had had diabetes for 17 years and played the "game" that many of us play . . . trying to project what my future health would be. I found it enormously uplifting to meet this woman. She was living proof that some people live very well with diabetes.

More than 20 years later, I was at the health club and noticed a young woman in her 20s using a blood glucose meter in the locker room. I commented: "I have one of those, too."

She said: "I have only recently been diagnosed."

I responded with that powerful sentence: "I've had diabetes for 41 years."

She exclaimed: "Oh, that's so encouraging!"

"I know," I said. "That's why I told you."

What if it truly doesn't matter what you do but how you do whatever you do? . . . .What if the question is not why am I so infrequently the person I really want to be, but why do I so infrequently want to be the person I really am?

—Oriah Mountain Dreamer

Adapt to the ongoing changes in your life. Applying this quotation to diabetes means that we don't have to like having diabetes. But, if we are to have a good quality of life, then we need to adapt to what is and deal constructively with the reality of having diabetes.

What helps you to adapt? Blood glucose monitoring? Education programs? Your health care team? Family, friends, coworkers? Your spirit?

When you meet a person who has inner authentic presence, you find he has an overwhelming genuineness, which might be somewhat frightening because it is so true and honest and real. You experience a sense of command radiating from the person . . . although that person might be a garbage collector or a taxi driver, still he or she has an uplifted quality, which magnetizes you and commands your attention.

—Chogyam Trungpa

Listen to your inner wisdom. Your health care team can give you essential information for managing diabetes, but only you can know what is essential for managing your life.

Listen to your own values, goals, and needs. Connect with all the resources you have to live according to your values. Meet your needs as only you can. Set your own goals. The goals you set are the only ones you will have the energy to pursue and achieve.

Listen to your true, authentic self.

The very least you can do in your life is to figure out what you hope for. And the most you can do is live inside that hope.

—Barbara Kingsolver

Integrate diabetes and life. Diabetes affects and is affected by all aspects of life. To become empowered we need to identify our goals and our problems and our resources. If quality of life (as defined by the individual) is the goal, and diabetes is the problem, then we identify all the external and inner resources to achieve our goals and overcome our problems. The outcome of this empowerment process is the integration of diabetes and life.

Diabetes cannot be left on the kitchen counter when we go shopping . . . or in the glove box when we pull into the employee parking lot . . . or in the bathroom when we leave on vacation.

Diabetes and life need to be integrated, so that diabetes gets managed and life gets enjoyed.

One of my colleagues once said: There are only four kinds of people in the world—those who have been caregivers, those who currently are caregivers, those who will be caregivers, and those who will need caregivers.

—Rosalynn Carter

Teach all of your supporters how they can support you. Friends need to understand why timing of meals is important when we use insulin. Family members need to understand what's going on with blood glucose if we are to receive their cooperation. Our health care team needs to know who we are and what we value if we are to truly form an effective team.

People cannot read our minds. Share, communicate, . . . teach.

Teach love, for that is what you are.

—George Eliot

Begin each day as if it were on purpose.
                              —Mary Ann Radmacher

Yes! Keep looking for everything that is YES around you and within you. Connect with all the stories, people, and experiences that ignite your spirit and affirm what you value about life. Seek quality. Build a quality life.

Question
　　Uplift
　　　　Adapt
　　　　　　Listen
　　　　　　　　Integrate
　　　　　　　　Teach
　　　　　　　　　　Yes!

Education is learning what you didn't even know you didn't know.

—Daniel J. Boorstin

Mental visualization is a powerful tool. Psychologists tell us that we move in the direction of our most dominant thought. Another spin on that idea is to say that "expectation becomes self-fulfilling prophecy." We expect something to happen. We visualize the outcome. We move in that direction because we have transformed the goal into a blueprint.

There is one more important dimension of reaching a goal through visualization—belief. We must believe what we can only see in our mind's eye.

I shared this concept of mental imagery once with a bank president. He planned to use it in his golf game. Some weeks later I gave a program for his employees, and I asked about his golf game. He said visualization had not worked for him, but, after hearing my presentation he knew why. "That's it! I visualized, but I didn't believe. I'd say to myself, 'That's where I want the ball to go, but it won't.' I visualized but didn't believe."

God made the sea, we make the ship; He made the wind, we make a sail; He made the calm, we make the oars.

—Senegal proverb

When people are able to move beyond the anger and denial that are quite natural responses to the diagnosis of diabetes, they stop placing blame and look within themselves for the strength and resources to live well with this challenge.

As is eloquently expressed in the Senegal proverb, we have a role to play, a responsibility, and an opportunity. The following affirmations come to mind as I meditatively read the Senegal proverb.

I have the responsibility for my life.

I have a blood glucose monitor; I will use it and act on the information.

I have a knowledgeable, caring health care team; I will see them regularly.

I have walking shoes; I will walk.

Just trust yourself, then you will know how to live.
—Johann Wolfgang von Goethe

Distraction is a helpful technique for pain management. Many have reported that a toothache has disappeared when the mind is distracted by a game, movie, or stimulating conversation. What is true for physical pain can also be true for mental and spiritual pain. Here are some distractions:

- novel that literally takes you away to another place and time
- movie that pulls you into its story from beginning to end
- telephone call or visit with someone who cares about you
- project in your house
- visit to the library to explore its offerings
- walk down the main street of a neighboring city
- meeting a friend for coffee in a new or favorite coffee shop

Make your own list, tape it to the inside of a cupboard door in your kitchen. When your summer spirit fizzles, go to your list for refreshment.

A man's capacity is the same as his breadth of vision.

—Arab proverb

Graduations, confirmations, baptisms, and bar mitzvahs—all of these signs of "passage" bring me to a card shop. And once again, I ponder the questions these cards raise and apply them to my own life.

When I read the hopeful wishes for graduates about who they will become, I ask myself who I have become. With the help of the poetry and lofty phrases on the cards, I review my own life.

Will you be ethical? Wise? Honest? Compassionate? Will you be smart so that you can make your way in this world? Will you give more than you take? What will you value above all else? Who will remember you? Why?

The same integrity that guides our direction at work, in our homes, and with our friends is the personal integrity that guides our choices in managing diabetes.

Integrity is a wholeness of the spirit that causes our whole life to be in agreement. Integrity occurs when what we say and what we do are the same.

Beauty is not caused. It is.

—Emily Dickinson

Apply that thought to joy. Joy is different from happiness, which can be caused. The causes for happiness are as many and as varied as there are people. We can be made happy because the weather is beautiful on a day we have planned a picnic or a bike ride. Happiness can be caused by an unending list of external factors that combine to provide us with what we think we want. While happiness is caused by outside circumstances, joy is a spiritual, inner quality.

While with an eye made quiet by the power of harmony, and the deep power of joy, we see into the life of things.

—William Wordsworth

Meditate on the joy in your life. What is its source? How do you access joy? Does your joy help you to "see into the life of things?"

Everybody wants to be somebody; nobody wants to grow.

—Goethe

A counselor told the story of meeting with a man whose life was totally out of control. His story included drugs, jail, and divorce. His body posture communicated his hopelessness.

The counselor said to him: "I see a boat being controlled by the swift current in the river. Wherever the current takes it, the boat goes. There are piles of jagged rocks in the river. The boat could crash."

The man quietly responded, "I see what you're saying."

"Look in the bottom of the boat," said the counselor. "What do you see?"

"Oars," was the man's response.

My blood glucose monitor and strips are the oars that I use to steer through the river of diabetes.

That is happiness; to be dissolved into something completely great.

—Willa Cather

A blessing that diabetes has provided me is the opportunity to meet many wonderful people who are affected by diabetes either because they have it, a loved one has it, or they are health care professionals. Together we have worked on raising funds for research and supporting the programs of the American Diabetes Association.

We have helped one another to grow, to heal, to laugh again. We have rallied around people newly diagnosed with diabetes. We have been the community activists to get political support for diabetes education and supplies. We have helped to inform the broader community about diabetes.

We have moved outside of ourselves and our worlds to dissolve into the larger concern for others.

We are what we consume. If we look deeply into the items that we consume every day, we will come to know our own nature very well.
                                    —Thich Nhat Hanh

Table graces are said by many people and represent a wide diversity of religious and cultural traditions. Most of them express gratitude for food about to be received as well as an acknowledgement of our role in giving back as we have received. As we are nourished, may we so nourish life.

A table grace has long been a family tradition for me. Some years after I was diagnosed with diabetes, I received a new insight from our table grace. When I focus on my gratitude for the food and my responsibility of returned service, eating has a new meaning. I don't eat because I have to meet my insulin. I don't eat just because I'm hungry or the food tastes good. I eat as part of my service to life.

Bless this food to our use and us to Thy service.

Be glad of life because it gives you the chance to love and to work and to play and to look at the stars.

—Henry Van Dyke

It is precisely because I am glad of life that I work at managing diabetes. Being "glad of life" can show itself in many ways. Basically, I see it as loving life itself. I experience this love standing in a field looking at the wildflowers, listening to the laughter of a small child, walking through my neighborhood appreciating with profound gratitude that I can walk . . . and I experience the gladness of life every morning when I awaken. "Thank you" are usually the first words I say.

I am reminded of the very first prayer our son said: "Thank you, God, another day!"

To see a World in a Grain of Sand
And a Heaven in a Wild Flower
Hold Infinity in the palm of your hand
And Eternity in an hour . . .

—William Blake

One need not be a poet to see the infinite in the finite. Look around you today. See the beauty in a flower, then go beyond simple beauty, and see the divine. It's there. Open yourself to see, to hear, to smell, to feel, to be.

Well, summer is almost over . . . There's never enough time to do all the nothing you want.
—Calvin and Hobbes

Consider engaging in a mental imagery exercise. Quiet yourself and sit in a place where you are unlikely to be disturbed. Close your eyes and focus on your breathing. Place your hand on your abdomen and feel your abdomen move as you breathe deeply. Spend several minutes like this, focused on your breathing, relaxing.

In your mind's eye travel to a favorite summer place . . . a cabin on a lake . . . a bonfire at the edge of the river . . . a backyard gazebo or porch . . . a park. Experience and enjoy this place with all of your senses. Recall the aroma of a fire, the sounds of a guitar, singing or laughter, feel a gentle breeze touching your face. Stay in this relaxing moment as long as you can and want to.

When you return by opening your eyes, do you feel more relaxed? Has this experience been helpful? What could you do next time to make the experience even better?

If you must play, decide upon three things at the start: the rules of the game, the stakes, and the quitting time.

—Chinese proverb

Clearly, all of us with diabetes must play, whether we want to or not, so it is wise for us to learn more about diabetes. We need to know how much we have to lose, and how to keep from losing it. We need to know what we owe diabetes today. The stakes, you know, are high. But if we do all we can to get our A1C down to 7 by choosing to eat wisely and to exercise every day, and by taking our medications on time, then we have the very best odds at beating the complications of diabetes. And we feel better and have more energy right now. You may not be able to quit, but you sure can rest easier when you play by the rules.

There are some people who have the quality of richness and joy in them and they communicate it to everything they touch. It is first of all a physical quality; then it is a quality of the spirit.

—Thomas Wolfe

I need those people in my life. Their spirit ignites mine.

Reflect on the people you know who have the quality that Wolfe describes. They are refreshment for our souls as surely as water quenches our thirst.

My friend Anne has that quality of richness and joy. Every time I see her (most often by chance in the grocery store), her face lights up with warmth and joy and love. That quality was not extinguished after her sister died. Nor after her mother died. Nor after her cancer surgery. This quality is not physical. It is a quality of the spirit.

Affirmation of life is the spiritual act by which man ceases to live unreflectively and begins to devote himself to his life with reverence in order to raise it to its true value. To affirm life is to deepen, to make more inward, and to exalt the will to live.
—Albert Schweitzer

I have based my work on the belief in three driving principles: Cope, Support, and Hope—the psychosocial/spiritual. In the mid-1980s, I wrote the following affirmations to accompany the seminar that I developed and still facilitate.

I will meet Life's challenges with a spirit of determination.

I will cope with Life's stresses, controlling what I can, and letting go of worry over stresses that I cannot control.

I will seek support whenever I need it. I will receive support gratefully and give it generously.

I will live Today well, remembering the lessons and happiness of Yesterday, and believing in the promises and hope of Tomorrow.

For today well-lived makes every yesterday a dream of happiness and every tomorrow a vision of Hope.
—Kalidasa

Music washes away from the soul the dust of everyday life.

—Berthold Auerback

Dust accumulates in our lives in the form of *routine*. That includes our management of diabetes. Meal plans become routine and boring. We get stuck in the same old menus, and when we no longer need to refer to a recipe or cookbook, it can be a sign that we're stuck in a rut. Sometimes novelty alone can be the spark that motivates us to follow a meal plan or exercise program. Books, magazines, classes, or even your health care professional can be the music that rekindles your soul.

At every turn in the road a new illumining is
needed to find the way and a new kindling is
needed to follow the way.

—John Dunne

High blood sugar can make you feel too tired to move. In fact, the tiredness is often what brings a person with not-yet diagnosed type 2 diabetes to the doctor. Diabetes is a turn in the road. To take good care of yourself and to bring those high blood sugars down, get up and take a walk. Today and tomorrow.

Only in growth, reform, and change, paradoxically enough, is true security to be found.
—Anne Morrow Lindbergh

Some people want to take the same medications without ever trying new ones because the medication has worked for them in the past and they feel secure in sticking with it. However, the story of diabetes is one of growth and change. Although yesterday's medications may still work, the new ones often work better. Change should not be engaged in just for the sake of change, but change should be considered whenever it is presented because it may lead to even greater security. Be certain that you have a health care professional with whom you feel secure so that you can discuss medications and any other issues affecting your health and well-being.

It's never too late—in fiction or in life—to revise.
—Nancy Thayer

Life has been described by numerous metaphors. Sometimes it is compared to a journey, and or even to a sporting event. Think of your life as if it were a novel, a story sitting in a computer. Which parts of your story would you like to revise? Although you can't rewrite what's already happened, new insights into your history can give you different feelings about it. If you can learn the lessons of your past, you have a better chance of revising the script for today and, thus, shaping tomorrow.

Since we cannot change reality, let us change the eyes which see reality.

—Nikos Kazantzakis

The events of our lives cannot be changed. But how we *view* the events can be changed. Aldous Huxley had a great perspective on this. He said, "Experience is not what happens to you; it's what you do with what happens to you." Diabetes can be viewed as a punishment, or it can be seen as an opportunity to live a healthy lifestyle. People with diabetes have competed in the Olympics and won gold medals; they've married, given birth, and lived happy, fulfilling lives. Half full? Half empty? The choice is yours.

The strongest principle of growth lies in human choice.

—George Eliot

*E*mpowerment may be an overused word, but it's a great concept. And choice is at the heart of empowerment. Each of us is personally responsible for the actions we take and for the choices we make. And when we embrace the idea that we are responsible for our lives, we become empowered. Growth and self-confidence are the rewards. Lest we become too serious in all of this, remember the immortal words of Winnie the Pooh:

I was going to change my shirt, but I changed my mind instead.

—A. A. Milne

Change is not merely necessary to life. It is life.
—Alvin Toffler

Some people thrive on change, whereas others look at the word and their stomach starts churning. Where are you on the continuum between loving change and dreading it? If you dread change, take the "Swiss cheese" approach. Take a big task (the change that confronts or confounds you) and break it down into many little tasks. See the task in your mind's eye as a big piece of Swiss cheese, full of holes because you have changed a big task into many small ones. Take on one at a time.

The way to get started is to quit talking and begin doing.

—Walt Disney

Talking can lead to problem solving. It can enlist someone's support. It can bring clarity to obstacles you face and help you make a plan for action. But there are times when talking takes the place of doing, when it becomes a way to avoid acting. The surest way to get started is to start *doing*. Just do it!

Teachers open the door, but you must enter by yourself.

—Chinese proverb

Each class, each appointment with a health care professional, is an opportunity to learn and to travel to a new place. But these opportunities represent responsibilities for the learner. The teacher can present the information; the learner decides whether or not to use it. Diabetes is not managed by health care professionals, it is managed by the people who have it.

Truth is eternal, knowledge is changeable. It is disastrous to confuse them.

— Madeleine L'Engle

There have been and continue to be many changes in what we know about diabetes and how it is best managed. Recommendations are made based upon the best knowledge available at the time. For instance, we used to urge daily soaking of one's feet. Now the advice is not to soak one's feet, because soaking dries the skin and breaks down the tissue. In the 1950s, people were advised to take one shot of insulin per day. The recommendation then went to three or four shots a day. Now we have insulin pumps, which mimic the pancreas's delivery of insulin even more closely. Information changes, and if we were to accept the knowledge of the 1950s as the "truth" and base our practices on that outdated knowledge, the impact on our health would indeed be disastrous.

Laughter is inner jogging.

—Norman Cousins

When we laugh, the brain releases endorphins. These chemicals are the body's natural painkillers and spirit boosters. Open yourself to sources of laughter. Seek them out each day.

Pain is deeper than all thought,
Laughter is higher than all pain.

—Elbert Hubbard

*Sometimes it's good to hush up a while and let
autumn stick in a few words.*

—Calvin to Hobbes

I love the Fall of the year! Crisp air, leaves aflame waving from the trees, and excited children heading to school. As I watch them walk toward the bus, I see their smiles. Their book bags will be full this afternoon when they get off the bus. Now they hold only shiny new crayons with a waxy aroma and blank notebooks awaiting the touch of young fingers and explorations of eager minds.

I envy the children. Life is new again each Fall. Then I receive an insight. Fall can be a new beginning, even now. In fact, each day I ride the school bus of life to the classroom of my heart. English can come from any of the books on my shelf. History in every building I visit, every person I meet. Diabetes has been an important teacher since I was diagnosed in 1957. I continue to learn about life and health, coping with challenges, giving of myself to help others, experiencing spiritual places, and receiving the love I find there. So, today, I board the school bus of life and eagerly anticipate the lessons I will receive.

People are usually more convinced by reasons they discovered themselves than by those found by others.
—Blaise Pascal

Exercise has been recommended for many years in order to keep our weight down, strengthen our cardiovascular system, manage our blood glucose levels, and simply because it's one of the things we need to do to manage our diabetes. However, people generally become convinced by the reasons they discover for themselves, such as:

- I feel better when I increase my daily activity, but I don't need to "exercise." I can just
  - walk the dog a little farther each time
  - dance to the music on the radio (in the privacy of my kitchen)
  - take 10-minute walks several times a day
  - pick up the pace when I walk
  - play with children or grandchildren
- I feel proud of myself when my HDL goes up and my weight comes down
- I feel better about myself, more confident.

Even if you hate to exercise, can you increase your activity level? Forget that long list of things you need to do first, all the reasons you can't do it today, and the never-ending excuses.

DOn't wa**IT.**

As one goes through life, one learns that if you don't paddle your own canoe, you don't move.
— Katharine Hepburn

In the old days, we were accustomed to being cared for by an all-knowing medical professional, who gave us medication designed to treat or even cure our ills. We, the patient, did not have to do much at all, and it promoted a sort of passivity in us. Then, chronic diseases like diabetes came along and changed all that. Today, patients themselves are learning to manage the disease . . . each day, sometimes every hour of the day.

If we want to be healthy, we paddle our own canoe.

*Don't consider losses a waste of time. Consider
them an apprenticeship.*
                    —Greg Norman, professional golfer

Athletes see losses as lessons. Scientists see
failed experiments in the same light. By studying what
does not work and why, they move closer to finding
what does work.

*When self-blood glucose monitoring first became
available, I monitored a lot, finding out what the
impact was of a variety of food. I especially enjoyed
my research at Dairy Queen.*

In calm waters, every ship has a good captain.
—Swedish proverb

If the oceans and waterways were always calm, good captains would not be valued; they would not even be necessary. When the metaphoric ocean of our lives becomes agitated and turbulent because of storms like diabetes, then we need to be very good captains of our ship. Diabetes education gives us the charts and radar to help us navigate through choppy waters and rolling seas. It also helps to know an "old salt" or two who have successfully navigated through diabetes. Sometimes they have good advice and can offer a lot of support.

Abraham Lincoln wrote a reflection on his son's first day of school. Of course, his words also apply to daughters, and, in fact, to us all. He knew his son was embarking on a great adventure that "probably will include wars and tragedy and sorrow."

> To live in this world will require faith and love and courage. So World, teach him the things he will have to know.
> Teach him that it is far more honorable to fail than to cheat.
> Teach him to sell his brawn and his brains to the highest bidders, but never to put a price tag on his heart and soul.

These are inspiring words, particularly so for us at John's baptism. They focused us on what we really value, to understand there is more to a child's life than an injury to his foot and leg.

I shared this thought with children with diabetes and their parents. I suggested we step back and see the whole picture—that there is more to life than diabetes. How interesting, though, that it is diabetes or injury that calls forth the faith, love, and courage. Is that what is meant by "a blessing in disguise?"

*The human race has one really effective weapon,
and that is laughter.*

—Mark Twain

Barbara Johnson, the "Geranium Lady," provides humor in her books as well as a helpful perspective on the value of laughter. "Laughter is the shock absorber that eases the potholes of life. Laughter is like premium gasoline; it helps take the knock out of living." A sense of humor is connected to the way you look at life . . . the way you put your problems in perspective. Laugher may not get you out of your tunnel, but it will definitely light your way.

Don't find fault. Find a remedy.

—Henry Ford

The blame game does no one any good. And it doesn't fix the problem. Whether building a car or a healthy body, seek solutions to problems. Here is a time-honored, four-step problem-solving model:

1. Stop. Take time to define the problem accurately.
2. Think of all the possible solutions you can and list them.
3. Act on one of the solutions.
4. Review and evaluate it. Is the problem solved? If so, great. If not, go back to the list of solutions and keep trying them until you have it solved.

To help you remember the process, think of the STAR approach. Stop, Think, Act, Review.

Sleep is the best meditation.

—The Dalai Lama

By learning how to manage stress, we can prevent it from causing serious problems. Here are some tips from *Diabetes Forecast* (July 2002):

- Get up earlier so you don't have to rush.
- Don't gulp lunch at your desk. Take a walk and enjoy a change of scenery. You'll be focused and accomplish more when you get back.
- When you start to feel overwhelmed, take a minute to breathe in and out slowly.
- Learn how to meditate and set aside time to do it two or three times a day.
- See a counselor who does cognitive and behavioral therapy. This kind of therapy zooms right to the heart of the problem. Together, you identify which of your ideas and behaviors worsens your stress, and you work on changing your *response* to the stress.
- Say "no" to demands on your time that would overload you. You then have more time for what really matters, such as family.
- Get a full night's sleep. Most people need 9 hours!
- Make time each week for activities you enjoy.

Fear makes the wolf bigger than he is.
—German proverb

Is there a "wolf" in your life? What is it? Or do you have a whole pack of wolves in your life right now? Sometimes, information is all that is needed to dispel fear. Talk with your diabetes educator and express your concerns. Ask questions. If you are still fearful, the cognitive therapy counseling approach can help cut the wolf down to size. Ask your diabetes educator about it.

Any fact facing us is not as important as our attitude toward it, for that determines our success or failure.

—Norman Vincent Peale

Star athlete Wilma Rudolph was taught by her mother that she could accomplish anything she wanted. She was born with a crippling disease, and her mother was told she would never walk. But her mother refused to believe this, scraping together the money for treatment. Wilma's first achievement was to walk without braces. She later went on to become the first woman to receive three gold medals in one Olympics, but it never would have happened if she hadn't believed that it could.

If you can't change your fate, change your attitude.
—Amy Tan

Another gem from the wisdom and humor of Barbara Johnson:

Things not to do when you're feeling blue:

Don't weigh yourself.
Don't watch "Old Yeller."
Don't go near a chocolate shop.
Don't open your credit card bill.
Don't go shopping for a new bathing suit.

Stress does not kill us so much as ingenious adaptation to stress facilitates our survival.
—George Vaillant, MD

We can adapt to the stress of diabetes by

- Eating nutritiously (eat premium fuel)
- Being active (dance, play, run, skip, clean, garden)
- Giving and receiving support (make friends and be good to your family)
- Learning about health and self (read, ask questions, take a class)
- Engaging in self-management (changing our behaviors that get in our way)
- Changing attitudes by changing thoughts (using your mind power for good)

What adaptations would you add to this list?

Thinking is the soul talking to itself.

—Plato

Monitor your thoughts. Just as blood glucose monitoring gives you helpful information for managing your diabetes, thought monitoring helps you manage yourself. Listen to your self-talk. What actions are likely to follow these thoughts? If the actions are not taking you in the direction you want to go, then change your thoughts. What is your treatment of choice for low blood sugar? What is your favorite means of raising your thoughts and mood?

Thought and learning are of small value unless translated into action.

—Wang Ming

How many diabetes classes, lectures, and events have you attended? How many diabetes books, magazines, articles, and web pages have you read? What have you *done* as a result of what you have learned? Each time you read or hear something about diabetes, make a decision about what you will *do* with that learning.

The [person] who removes a mountain begins by carrying away small stones.

—Chinese proverb

List the "mountains" you encounter in your experience with diabetes. The diagnosis itself can seem to be a monumental obstacle. Weight loss can appear to be a huge challenge, and maintaining an exercise program is another mountain to climb. Set a few small goals—some foothill goals. After achieving them, set a few more. As you see progress in reaching your goals, record the step-by-step transformation of each mountain-sized challenge into a pile of stones. *Celebrate!*

Obstacles are what we see when we take our eyes off our goal.

—Howard Hendricks

Instead of having a vague idea of what your goal is, define and describe it in detail. Is your goal a trim, healthy body? Do you have a picture of yourself looking like that? If so, make copies of it and put the picture everywhere: desk, refrigerator, dash board, inside your checkbook, places where you will see it daily. Keep your eyes on your goal.

It's not by doing the things we like, but by liking the things we do that we can discover life's blessings.

—Goethe

Are there positive aspects to the lifestyle of diabetes? How can diabetes be thought of as a "blessing in disguise"? What are some of the things you would say to someone newly diagnosed with diabetes?

Learn to get in touch with the silence within yourself and know that everything in this life has a purpose, there are no mistakes, no coincidences, all events are blessings given to us to learn from.

—Elisabeth Kubler-Ross

The gem cannot be polished without friction, nor man perfected without trials.

—Confucius

We cannot choose which trials we will encounter in life. We do choose how we will handle them. This process begins with thinking, because thoughts guide and direct our behavior. What thoughts do you have about diabetes? Is this philosophy of Confucius one that you can easily embrace? Does it help you accept that you have diabetes? If not, look for thoughts that fit comfortably into your belief system.

You win not by chance but by preparation.
—Roger Maris

Baseball great Roger Maris knew how to win baseball games. But this wisdom goes well beyond baseball. Winning at life requires preparation. People who have diabetes prepare for "winning" by having their blood glucose monitor with them at all times. They check before and after working out, before taking insulin, before driving a car, and before bedtime. Preparation may also include keeping a pair of sneakers in the trunk so that a bit of extra time in one's day can be spent walking! Keeping some form of carbohydrate handy to treat a low is another way to be prepared. What others come to mind?

It is the ability to choose which makes us human.
—Madeleine L'Engle

Our choices are influenced by outside forces, like movies, advertising, family tradition, friends, and coworkers. But our choices are guided by internal forces as well: *values, beliefs, hopes, and goals.*

Choose well the food you eat, the activity you include in your life, and the methods you use to manage stress—and remember that doing nothing is also a choice. Healthy choices move us toward good health.

I like spring, but it is too young. I like summer, but it is too proud. So I like best of all autumn; because its leaves are a little yellow, its tone mellower, its colors richer. And it is tinged a little with sorrow. Its golden richness speaks not of the innocence of spring, nor of the power of summer, but of the mellowness and kindly wisdom of approaching age. It knows the limitations of life and is content.
—Lin Yutang

Reconnect with the wisdom you already have, the wisdom that has always been and always will be inside of you. Different from knowledge that changes with each new piece of information, wisdom is lasting and universal truth. Wisdom is profound and changeless.

Reflect on the wisdom found in family stories, proverbs, your ever-developing philosophy of life, observations of world thought leaders, and your experience with life.

Knowledge is proud that he has learned so much;
Wisdom is humble that he knows no more.
—William Cowper

Knowledge about diabetes has changed and continues to change. Years ago, we were told to soak our feet every day in water to which we added soap. Now we are told that daily soaking breaks down tissue, and soap is too drying. In other words, the new advice is: Don't soak your feet! Recommendations about insulin have changed from multiple injections (when we only had regular) to one shot (when intermediate-acting insulin was discovered) back to multiple injections following the DCCT and UKPDS.

As knowledge changes, wisdom keeps our minds open to new information and the ongoing changes in therapies and lifestyle recommendations. Without this wisdom, we may view change as a frustrating betrayal of our trust in medicine and health care professionals. Wisdom kindly grants a fresh perspective and helps us accept change.

Zeal without knowledge is fire without light.
—Thomas Fuller

The truth is that we must be enthusiastic, even zealous, about taking care of our diabetes and be sincerely committed to doing so—and we need to be educated about how to do that. Are you regularly updating your diabetes knowledge and skills and learning how to manage it?

Even blood glucose monitoring skills are improved by a check of technique with a diabetes educator. There may be a new meter that meets your needs better, too!

A Native American elder once described his own inner struggles in this manner: "Inside of me there are two dogs. One of the dogs is mean and evil. The other dog is good. The mean dog fights the good dog all the time." When asked which dog wins, he reflected for a moment and replied, "The one I feed the most."

—George Bernard Shaw

Dr. Clarissa Pinkola Estes, author of *Women Who Run with the Wolves* and *The Gift of Story* refers to stories as medicine. She notes that "Tales, legends, myths, and folklore are learned, developed, numbered, and preserved the way a pharmacopoeia is kept. A collection of cultural stories, and especially family stories, is considered as necessary for long and strong life as decent food, decent relationships, and decent work." She informs us that in her family the telling of stories is an essential spiritual practice.

What are the stories you have heard around the kitchen or dining room table? What do you know about yourself based on family stories? What strengths have people in your family shown through their life stories? Many families have "horror" stories. What are your family's "healing" stories? Tell them. Again and again.

Happiness is a how, not a what; a talent, not an object.

—Herman Hesse

Throughout our lives we develop a philosophy (or a series of them). One purpose I have in writing this book is to encourage you to become aware of and develop a helpful philosophy, one that will give meaning to your lives and help you live comfortably with your experiences.

Philosophy can seem obscure at times, but its value is in getting us to think. Consider the following story and the meaning it holds for you.

A familiar philosophy is found in the adage: "If Life gives you lemons, make lemonade. Do the best with what you've been given." I have found that philosophy useful at times, but trite and irritating at other times in my life. I received a great insight into my personal philosophy when I heard a pastor say from the pulpit: "If life gives you lemons and you don't like lemonade, then throw the lemons back and demand strawberries!"

The original philosophy was missing the important element of choice. If I don't like lemonade, I don't have to make it. We do have choices.

Those who would rightly understand someone must first read the whole story.

—A proverb

Support is an important part of life and of living well with diabetes. For health care professionals to support us, they must understand who we are. For many years, diabetes education focused on the disease instead of on the person. But, diabetes is managed, must be managed, by the person who has it every day.

In 2003 at the International Diabetes Federation (IDF) meeting in Paris, Dr. Urban Rosenquist reported on his research in diabetes education. He said programs that focus on the person (history, culture, family) are more effective in managing diabetes than programs that focus on diabetes.

Does your health care team know who you are? Do they understand the forces that have shaped you—your personal history, cultural influences past and present? Tell them your story and update it at each visit. Diabetes is a process, changed by and changing with the life experiences of the people who have it.

We all walk in the dark. And it is up to each one of us to turn on our own light.
— Katharine Hepburn

At a diabetes conference Dr. Jean Philippe Assal of the University of Geneva, Switzerland showed a slide of a lovely pastoral scene. But, it had a big "blob" in the middle, almost as if a drop of paint had fallen on the canvas by mistake. His comment was: "Diabetes is a rupture on the landscape of people's lives." Dr. Assal's comment was a compassionate recognition of the impact that diabetes has in the lives of people who have it. He was speaking to physicians and reaching them with an important message about the human implication of diabetes.

Consider how diabetes has disrupted your life. Share your insights with your health care team. They can help coach you through the "rupture" of diabetes.

Seek opportunities to meet other people who have diabetes. They can be an excellent resource for coaching and supporting you through rough times.

The rift in the chest of a mountain
The twist in the trunk of a tree,
The water-cut cave in the hollow,
The rough, rocky rim of the sea. . .
Each one has a scar of distortion,
Yet each has this sermon to sing,
"The presence of what would deface me,
Has made me a beautiful thing."

—Anonymous

As you travel through life, you will find new philosophies that can change your feelings toward diabetes—or any challenge you face. You may have already discovered that your experience with diabetes has made you empathetic with other people who have challenges. You may see strengths in yourself that were not visible until diabetes called on them. Are there blessings to be found in diabetes? When I left home my mother sent me this poem that answers that question for me.

A man is but a product of his thoughts; what he thinks, that he becomes.

—Mohandas K. Gandhi

Words can release stress and restore feelings of peace. How? By promoting mental images that relax and rejuvenate us.

FLOAT is a word that reminds me to relax. I think about being in the water at the beach, facing large waves, and choosing not to struggle but, instead, to float. I see a feather or a leaf gently floating through the air. Both the feather and the leaf whisper their healing message and timeless wisdom: Float.

We know that mental images are powerful tools in stress management. But just when we need them the most, when we are under the greatest stress, we find it difficult to get the soothing image on the projection screen of our minds. That's why words are so helpful. Can you say the word "elephant" without seeing one?

Identify the words that bring healing, restorative images. Say them.

Growth demands a temporary surrender of security.

—Gail Sheehy

Life's lessons are everywhere, wisdom ever available. In my first experience with snorkeling, I learned two lessons—one philosophical, one practical. It was a windy day, and the water was choppy. With my mask in place, I could look at the surface disturbance and then look below the surface and see the calm watery world, the beauty untouched by surface winds. I immediately connected with the idea that surface irritations in life can distract us from the deeper issues. As I mused about needing to let go of superficiality to grasp the deeper meaning and beauty in life, I was vaguely aware that my lips felt numb.

Ignoring the numbness and writing it off to a tight-fitting mask, I continued my snorkeling reverie until I swam over a jellyfish and got stung. This sent me back to the mother ship for first aid. Once aboard, I decided to check my blood glucose. It was 40. My numb lips should have warned me about low blood sugar. How humbling.

Lesson number two: Don't get so absorbed in the meaning and beauty of a coral reef that you miss the obvious signs of hypoglycemia. Amen.

Habits are at first cobwebs, then, cables.
—Spanish proverb

Habit is a cable; we weave a thread of it every day, and at last we cannot break it.
—Horace Mann

A man is a slave to whatever has mastered him.
—II Peter 2:19

We are what we repeatedly do. Excellence, then, is not an act, but a habit.
—Aristotle

We first make our habits, and then our habits make us.
—John Dryden

Habits can be very helpful; for example, blood glucose monitoring that becomes as much a daily habit as tooth-brushing. Habits can be destructive when they involve smoking, drinking, or eating to manage stress. Make a list of some of the habits you are aware of in your life. What are the threads you weave daily? Are you a slave to any activity or routine? What is it that you repeatedly do? What healthy habits could you repeatedly do? Then, what would they make you?

Hope, like the gleaming tapers light,
Adorns and cheers our way;
And still, as darker grows the night,
Emits a brighter ray.

—Oliver Goldsmith

As you move through diabetes barriers and challenges toward the goals you hold in your heart, keep in mind:

FAITH
HOPE
CLARITY

Have faith. Hold tightly to your faith. Know the source of your faith and reconnect with your spiritual roots regularly.

Have hope. Revisit the cherished stories that keep the flame of hope burning.

Have clarity. Be clear about who you are, what you want, and where you are going. Good advice from your health care team is your map. A blood glucose meter is your compass. It is you who decide on your destination. With faith, hope, and clarity, you are more likely to get there and reap the rewards of a full life.

It is only possible to live happily ever after on a day to day basis.
—Margaret Bonnano

Just as our ancestors had to tend to the fire to keep their families warm, fed, and protected, so must we tend to our individual, inner fire. Managing diabetes day after day gets wearying and, sometimes, discouraging, when our results are different from what we had hoped. It is our inner fire that renews life energy or enthusiasm (literally defined as God within). Fuel for that inner fire comes in many forms. Consider these and make your own list.

- worship services
- music and other arts
- friends and the experience of friendship
- service to others
- prayer
- giving our unique gifts to help others
- meaningful work (including volunteer work)
- vacations
- inspiring reading with time to reflect and absorb

What have you done recently that fanned the flames of your inner fire? What do you have planned for the near future? Which activities are ongoing?

Don't let this be left up to chance. Tend to your fire.

We are the clay, and thou art our potter; we are all the work of thy hand.

—Isaiah 64:8

In the December 1997 *Diabetes Forecast* magazine, Dr. Robert Tattersall of England made this observation: "Technology has greatly improved the lives of people with diabetes, but it is clearly not a cure-all." Quoting Nobel Prize winner George Minot, Tattersall agreed that what is needed is to "teach the art of courageous living."

Great art conceals great art. The breathtaking beauty of ballet conceals the sweat and aching muscles that went into making the dance look effortless. Whether the artist is dancing, painting, playing music, or throwing pots, there is "art" hidden in the creation of the visible product. This hidden art is the artist's energy, devotion, and skill.

Courageous living is an art, not a science. There are no formulas or recipes. We create by doing. We create a courageous life by trusting, believing, and working hard with the gift of life that we have been given. Most likely, the only visible sign is the life itself. But in moments of quiet reflection, we are aware of the invisible beauty in it—the spiritual dimension—and the Artist's genius.

"What day is it?"
"It's today," squeaked Piglet.
"My favorite day," said Pooh.

—A.A. Milne

Cars, appliances, watches, radios—lots of things come to us with guarantees. We easily and understandably develop an expectation for guarantees in all of life . . . even for Life itself. Life comes with no guarantees.

We learned that when the diagnosis of diabetes was made. But that didn't end our expectation of some guarantee. When we know people who have lived 50 and 60 years with diabetes, we claim that expectation of longevity. Then we hear of someone who had a heart attack before age 30 or 40.

And, we learn, again, that we have no guarantees about life.

The blessing in what could be a frightening and frustrating situation is the recognition that life, each day, each moment, is precious. Thus blessed, we stop living in the tomorrow that no one is promised. We live today.

And, if we are truly wise, we LIVE today . . . each day.

Look, I really don't want to wax philosophic. But, I will say that if you're alive, you've got to flap your arms and legs, you've got to jump around a lot, you've got make lots of noise, because life is the very opposite of death!

—Mel Brooks

In the opening ceremony of the 1988 IDF meeting in Sydney, Australia, a doctor quoted from Shakespeare's *Julius Caesar*:

The fault, dear Brutus, lies not in our stars, but in ourselves . . . .

Read meditatively and apply this thought to your life. Do you see where the opposite could also be true? Our "answers" lie not outside of us, but within us? Do you have personal qualities that make diabetes management difficult? What are the personal qualities that help you meet the challenges of managing diabetes?

Faults may lie within us but so do answers.

The meaning of life is to find your gift,
the purpose of life is to give it away.

—Joy J. Golliver

In his poem *Psalm of Life*, Henry Wadsworth Longfellow reminds us that we leave behind us "footprints on the sand of time." Further, he suggests that our footprints can be the encouragement for a lost traveler to keep going.

Have you ever felt that you are alone in the challenges you face? Remember how good it felt to find people you believe have truly walked in the same moccasins? Now it is your footprints that can guide and inspire those who come after you. You leave footprints in the example you set by how you live.

Dr. Hans Selye was a Montreal physician who said that when we help others we help ourselves. We receive a lift by lifting up someone else.

The credit belongs to the man who is actually in the arena, whose face is marred by dust and sweat and blood, who strives valiantly, who errs and comes short again and again. Who knows the great enthusiasms, the great devotions, and spends himself in a worthy cause. Who at best knows achievement and who at least fails while daring greatly so his place shall never be with those cold and timid souls who know neither victory nor defeat.

—Theodore Roosevelt

A scholar who had studied Nobel Prize winners shared a remarkable story. He said that all Nobel Prize winners share one unanimously common characteristic: they had all reached a point in their work where they believed they had to give up. Obviously, they shared one more characteristic: they did not give up. Their Nobel Prizes are testimony to the fact that they continued to work.

Winston Churchill adds another dimension to this characteristic by applying it to living with a chronic disease. Most of his life, Churchill struggled with manic depression. This insight into his life makes his famous speech to a group of school children even more inspiring. His ten-word speech was: *Never give up. Never give up. Never, never, never, never.*

I always knew that one day I would take this road but yesterday I did not know today would be the day.

—Nagarjuna

In one of his most famous poems, Robert Frost speaks of how taking the road less traveled had made all the difference. Frost was writing about the choices we make and how our choices determine not only the direction but also the quality of our lives.

The experience each of us has with diabetes is largely of our choosing. Each day, each hour of each day, we choose our thoughts and, therefore, our attitudes. We choose our behaviors and experience their consequences. Diabetes "happened." What will you do with it?

Experience is not what happens to you; it is what you do with what happens to you.

—Aldous Huxley

You don't get to choose how you're going to die. Or when. You can only decide how you're going to live. Now.

— Joan Baez

At dinner one evening years ago, my husband told me about a new retirement plan for us. Suddenly, I heard myself say, "What? So you can spend it with some cute little blond?" We were both stunned by my uncharacteristic outburst. We finished dinner in a reflective silence.

Days passed, and I took the opportunity to reflect on that scene. I thought about what had happened recently. A diabetic friend of mine had just died at the age of 34 from complications of diabetes. She had graduated Phi Beta Kappa in pharmacy. She had two goals in life: to get married and to get a job. She died without realizing either goal.

Once again I had to come to grips with the loss of a young friend and the reality of my own mortality. At the same time, there was the realization that I am very healthy and have a good chance of living well into retirement. And, the experience connected me once again to my faith. I can only do so much, then I must let go and have faith.

Having come to this awareness and resolution, I shared it with my husband. Then I said, "I don't know about the cute or the little . . . but I have figured out how to stay blond."

Theatre is not about theatre; it is about life.
—Bertolt Brecht

The same can be said of diabetes (or any other chronic disease). For those of us who have it, our interest centers around the meaning diabetes has for daily living and overall satisfaction with life. What impact will diabetes have on my daily life? How will diabetes affect my ability to engage fully in an active and fulfilling life?

Sometimes health care professionals get caught up in the medical meaning of diabetes. Their response to the question: "What does diabetes mean?" may center on glucose metabolism.

I am grateful for my mother's answer that diabetes meant I would live a healthier, more disciplined life. When I asked her what diabetes meant, I was not looking for a scientific or medical response. I wanted her to tell me about me. She helped me to believe that I could always participate fully in life.

Diabetes is not about diabetes; it is about life.

God gave us memories so that we might have roses in December.

—Sir James Barrie

How does one keep roses well into December? One woman said that she finds it a real boost to keep photographs from vacations in a photo album so that she can revisit the places, cherish the memories. Another person described how enjoyable and uplifting a weekly coffee club has become. He said that members of the group share stories of their families, their vacations, their experiences . . . to be enjoyed again and again. The story was fresh in June, fun to remember in December!

An elderly woman who is blind made this insightful comment: "One should always furnish one's mind well. When I am alone, I can enjoy sitting in a well-furnished mind."

If there is anything we wish to change in a child, we should first see if it is not something that could better be changed in ourselves.

—Carl Jung

When my nephew Scott died, his wife, Sheila, was 30 years old, and their daughter, Maggie, was six months old. Sheila's friends said to her, "What a pity that Maggie will never know her daddy." Others said, "In the long run, it will be better for Maggie that she simply never even knew Scott."

Sheila's remarkable response to her friends was, "Look, it doesn't matter whether it's 'good' or 'bad.' It's the way it is."

I found other ways to apply this universal truth. Years ago when I spoke to audiences of people who have diabetes, I spoke to them as if I were a cheerleader selling them on the healthy lifestyle that diabetes requires. But it really doesn't matter whether people find the lifestyle requirements to be good or bad. *It's the way it is.* The task for each person is to figure out how to deal constructively with the reality of diabetes.

We all may have come on different ships, but we're in the same boat now.
—Martin Luther King, Jr.

A diabetes educator in Hawaii told me that the first thing in appointments with patients who have diabetes is that they "talk story." This is the ancient and important practice of conversation, of sharing-the-self, of connecting.

How insightful of Hawaiian practitioners to realize that they are dealing with whole people and cannot focus only on the physical aspects of diabetes. Blood vessels, organs, and nerves do not get diabetes. People do. Whole, intricate, complex human beings. In the process of telling our stories, we gain insights into who we are, and we share that insight with the people who can help us weave diabetes into our lives.

This practice might be Hawaiian, but it sounds broader than that. It sounds human. As a storyteller, an experience I always have when I tell stories is that people want to tell theirs.

We are all storytellers. Others' stories are how we learn of the universality of the human experience. We realize that we can and should "talk story" not only in Hawaii but also in Vermont and Mississippi and Arizona and Oregon.

Using urine testing results to manage diabetes is like driving a car by looking in the rearview mirror. All you know is where you've been.
—Dr. Sanford Smith

Dr. Smith's remark made me laugh with delight at a creative, wise description of the old way of testing glucose in urine. As I considered this comment further, I felt thankful for the progress I have experienced in the more than 40 years that I have had diabetes. Because of blood glucose monitoring, I can know where I am and can make wise decisions for moving forward in a positive direction . . . safely and comfortably. Actually, I prefer driving a car by looking forward through the windshield.

Knowledge is not power, it is only potential power that becomes real through use.

—Dorothy Riley

Consider the following statement:

I know how to monitor my blood glucose. I know how to adjust my food and exercise to keep blood glucose balanced. I know when I can handle diabetes management, and I know when I need to call my health care team for help. I know a lot about diabetes and its management. But, if I do not act on that knowledge, I am no better off than the person who knows nothing.

Would you describe this statement as true or false? Why? How do these thoughts apply to you?

To ask well is to know much.

—African proverb

To gain knowledge we must ask questions. Because we live better with diabetes when we know how to manage it, we need to consider how to ask questions well. That's why many of us write down our questions before each health care appointment. Some clinics even have forms they give out to patients to help them identify the questions they need answered.

Consider your questions. Do they get to the heart of the real issues? Is your question about the amount of fat in your meal plan reflecting a deeper concern about the amount of fat in your blood . . . and your family's history of heart disease? Perhaps "asking well" includes asking more completely. Complete questions include those issues that have to do with the physical concerns (Which protein source is lowest in fat?) as well as mental and spiritual concerns (How can I avoid being so worried about my heart?).

Ask well. Know much. Live better.

Who you are is where you were when.

That is the title of a training film used in the business world. It speaks to how we are shaped by our culture. Those of us who grew up during the 1950s were constantly reminded to eat all of our food because there were starving children in China. Being a member of the "clean plate club" was a great virtue.

Then, diabetes became part of who we are.

Living well with diabetes requires that our various cultural influences are carefully considered in terms of their impact on our diabetes management. Is it useful to belong to the clean plate club? (Was it ever?) What are today's cultural influences on your eating?

What are the cultural messages in your life today? How do they influence you?

A sailor without a destination cannot hope for a favorable wind.

—Leon Tec, MD

Sailboats crisscross, back and forth across the water, sometimes with the wind and sometimes against it. Their approach to sailing is very similar to a successful approach to diabetes management.

Sailors do not fight the wind, neither do they ignore it and hope that it will simply blow itself into the sail and move the boat. They understand the wind, and they have skills in sailing. They use their knowledge and experience to their advantage. They catch the wind through skilled techniques and make it work for them.

What do we do with blood glucose? Like wind providing the fuel for a sailboat, blood glucose provides the "fuel" for our bodies . . . if we use our knowledge, skill, and experience.

I discovered I always have choices, and sometimes it's only a choice of attitude.

—Abraham Lincoln

Two ladies were talking about a similar experience they have going to their respective church circles. Their views of their experiences led them to different choices and attitudes. One lady said, "I just hate going to my church circle. They always have some luscious dessert and they give me a piece of fruit. I feel so 'singled out'!"

To which her friend responded: "Really? My circle serves gooey desserts, but they give me whatever fruit is in season. That makes me feel so special!"

A strong positive mental attitude will create more miracles than any wonder drug.

—Patricia Neal

Dr. Viktor Frankl wrote Man's Search for Meaning drawing on his experiences as a psychiatrist and a survivor of Nazi concentration camps. Frankl believed that "decisions, not conditions" are what mental health is about. He also felt strongly that people do not get better by seeing themselves as a victim.

Some questions to consider: If diabetes is the condition, then what are the decisions that we can make to achieve mental health? The second question is: Do you see yourself as a victim or a victor?

Listen to your self-talk. What are the messages that you give yourself? Would you characterize them as being more life-affirming? Or self-defeating?

Finally, what decision can you make that will help you to see yourself as a victor?

A bad messenger plunges men into trouble, but a faithful envoy brings healing.

—Proverbs 13:17

A diabetes educator recalled meeting with a man newly diagnosed with diabetes. The man told the educator that he knew all about diabetes, about the complications he would experience, about his early death. His wife cried.

The startled educator asked him where he had learned about diabetes. He showed her a book that had been written 30 years earlier. The educator immediately began an up-to-date education that was, of course, far more hopeful.

Education is a never-ending process. We need to make sure that we have good resources for our education.

Something we were withholding made us weak
until we found out that it was ourselves.

—Robert Frost

A diabetes educator friend of mine told me that keeping a journal is the way that she discovers her spiritual self. She said that the journal is the place we realize how consistently we spin out the same webs only to be re-caught in them.

What an interesting thought! Is the spinning of a web similar to the setting of a goal? Have you ever set a goal (weight loss, regular exercise, meditative reading) only to find yourself re-setting that goal some weeks or months later? That's what getting "re-caught" in the same webs means to me.

Identify a goal that you set for yourself in the past year. If you did not reach the goal, explore why. Why do you find yourself re-caught in the same web? What will you do differently this time so you can achieve the goal?

Most of what I really need to know about how to live, and what to do, and how to be, I learned in kindergarten.

—Robert Fulghum

When his cat had kittens, my friend Bob learned food is comforting. Bob's mother gave all the children chocolate sundaes the day the kittens were given away. As an adult, Bob was very overweight. He realized that whenever he felt stressed, he ate. So, he chose exercise as a stress manager, instead.

Around the time I heard this story, my 4-year-old son, John, and I were shopping and became separated. When we finally found each other, we had a tearful reunion, and I bought him a cookie. As he put the cookie up to his sweet little mouth, I realized, with horror, that I was teaching my son the same thing. From then on, I avoided food as a comfort and a reward.

When our dog died, I called a neighbor and we told "Max" stories, laughing at the memories, crying over his loss . . . all the while healing. I hugged my son and told him what had helped me. There are healthy ways to manage stress. Max fathered 13 puppies. John knows where they are. Max's grandson could be in our future.

True listening brings us in touch even with that which is unsaid and unsayable.

—John O'Donohue

My Canadian grandmother read tea leaves. Nana could predict when she would get company and what the weather was likely to be.

I practice a more common reverie; I read clouds. The reading of clouds is not for predictions of future events. Reading clouds can be an enjoyable way to pass an hour or two on a summer afternoon or a pleasant, relaxing way to engage in the important act of self-reflection. And, because we gaze heavenward when we watch clouds, this could also be an opportunity for meditation—that is, listening to what God is saying to us.

Take time. Quiet yourself. Listen.

*Life is not a matter of holding good cards. It's
playing a poor hand well.*
　　　　　　　　　　　　　—Robert Louis Stevenson

Robert Louis Stevenson had tuberculosis most
of his life. His philosophy for living with a chronic
disease can be seen in his statement above. Each of us
decides how to play our cards. The experience of
having diabetes is largely of your own choosing.

The experience can be of deprivation and difficulty. The experience can be of growth and healthful
living. We choose our actions and our attitudes. What
are your actions and attitudes when you are playing
the hand of diabetes well?

Angels fly because they take themselves lightly.
　　　　　　　　　　　　　—G. K. Chesterton

We don't receive wisdom; we must discover it for ourselves after a journey that no one can take for us or spare us.

—Marcel Proust

The Search Institute in Minneapolis has done research into the personal assets that young people need to avoid high-risk behaviors. Our search is for the personal assets we need to live well with the challenge of diabetes. Research and personal experience have led me to believe that these traits include:

A positive attitude
The ability to solve problems
A positive self-image
Faith in a higher power
Healthy stress management
The capacity to adapt
Self-discipline
Motivation
Hope

What are the assets that have helped you? How did you discover them?

OCTOBER 29

There is only one thing more painful than learning from experience and that is not learning from experience.

—Archibald McLeish

A scientist looks at every experiment as a lesson from which to learn. When an experiment doesn't work, the scientist may say, "I tried. It didn't work, but I learned something." This leads to a philosophy that there is no failure, only lessons.

When I received my first blood glucose meter, I experimented by having an ice cream cone . . . dipped in chocolate. The resulting blood glucose was well over 200. I learned. Each day I am my own personal scientist . . . learning, one experiment at a time.

Wisdom comes to us lesson by lesson.

Quiet minds cannot be perplexed or frightened but go on in fortune or misfortune at their own private pace like the ticking of a clock during a thunderstorm.

—Robert Louis Stevenson

Our busy lives, daily stresses, and concerns often produce a mental state in us that is anything but quiet. Yet, most of us know that peace of mind is highly desirable. Once in a while, we experience peace that settles on us like the afghan Grandma used to throw over us when we were napping on the sofa. More often, to experience peace of mind, we must seek it. The Psalms are full of peace. Consider this thought:

Wait for the Lord; be strong, and let your heart take courage.

—Psalm 27:14

Wait for the Lord; be strong, and let your heart take
Wait for the Lord; be strong, and let your heart
Wait for the Lord; be strong, and let your
Wait for the Lord; be strong, and let
Wait for the Lord; be strong, and
Wait for the Lord; be strong,
Wait for the Lord; be strong,
Wait for the Lord; be
Wait for the Lord;
Wait for the
Wait for
Wait

When we fully rely upon the Lord to handle a given situation, He may, in his ultimate wisdom, remove all the obstacles and smooth out our path thoroughly. Or He may choose, instead, to walk with us along the rocky path.

—Charles R. Swindoll

Sometimes people say they are really counting on a cure for diabetes in their lifetime. Most of us hope for one. All of us would welcome it. But, counting on a cure can be dangerous if it means that you don't manage your diabetes now. During 40 years of diabetes, my position has been to manage it to the best of my ability so that when a cure does become available, I will be in the best possible health. I'll be ready!

In the book *Active Spirituality*, Charles R. Swindoll offers insight into what happens when people pray for a cure. His words provide comfort. Even if a cure is not found in our lifetime, we will not walk the rocky path of diabetes alone.

Picture a piece of embroidery placed between you and God, with the right side up toward God. Man sees the loose, frayed ends; but God sees the pattern.

—Corrie ten Boom

Life's mysteries may defy our understanding, but still we seek meaning. That's where philosophy, faith, and the arts come into play in our lives. We may never understand why we got diabetes, but we can find meaning in our experience with it.

Practical lessons that diabetes can teach us include the importance of goal setting, problem solving, and stress management. Spiritual meaning can come from a multitude of sources. Corrie ten Boom, author and survivor of the Holocaust, explained how she thinks about problems in life that defy understanding.

How can a thread like diabetes add to the beauty of Life's tapestry?

Shared sorrow is sorrow cut in half; shared joy is doubled.

—Swedish proverb

The daughter of a friend of mine has a handicapped child. When he was born, his handicap was a total surprise and a great shock. I wrote her a letter and shared all that I have to share, my heart. In part, the letter said:

"I believe that pain is never totally erased. We keep transcending it by God's grace and love. This love is expressed through family, friends, other families who share the same or similar challenge . . . and at some truly remarkable point, we begin to receive His power and love by *giving* it to others. That is the greatest blessing and, I believe, the sign that healing is really occurring. You can't rush the process. TRUST that you will get to that healing that allows you to transcend pain. God bless you with strength, love, laughter, tears, comfort, wisdom, power, and joy as you travel on your journey."

The gift is not how much you are loved, the gift is how much you are able to love.

—Unknown

Our efforts to "get over" the tragic events of life are misspent. These events shape us and the way we view life. Once we have experienced tragedy, it becomes a thread in the fabric of our life. However, we can choose whether that thread strengthens or weakens our fabric.

Our task is to find the meaning these experiences hold for us and use their lessons to heal ourselves and others. In observing people who have experienced tragedy, I have seen a common characteristic in the ones who make the most progress in healing. They focus on love instead of loss. Their "fabric" becomes stronger as their love strengthens others.

Dave spends a day a week volunteering at the hospital where his son, Scott, died. Jean, whose daughter, Julie, died, writes a book with her pastor on spiritual issues in adolescents' lives. Linda and Rich, who lost their daughter, Laura, build a healing garden . . . for the whole community.

Reflect on your response to tragedy. It's not too late to move toward love.

Do not be a slave to life's machinery; get a beautiful song, a lovely poem, and the whisper of God into your soul.

—Norman Vincent Peale

The pace of life seems to be a major source of stress for many of us. Even people who have retired talk about being too busy . . . too much to do . . . never enough time. The late Norman Vincent Peale wrote a lovely essay on "Taking Time to Live" and gave the advice above.

Do you have resources that give you spiritual nourishment? Look in the basement, the attic, or on your bookshelves. Many of us have books that we haven't read in some time. I am so grateful that I hung on to my textbooks in American, English, and world literature. Even things I've read before offer new insights—an unexpected beauty.

Let us be grateful to people who make us happy; they are the charming gardeners who make our souls blossom.

—Marcel Proust

If a man does not keep pace with his companions, perhaps it is because he hears a different drummer. Let him step to the music he hears, however measured or far away.

—Henry David Thoreau

An article in the *Harvard Business Review* titled "Management by Whose Objectives?" gave me an insight into diabetes management. The business community has long realized that the corporate goal will be achieved if individuals are allowed to set and achieve *their own* goals.

The corporate goal for diabetes is well-managed diabetes for everyone. To achieve that goal, we who have diabetes must be able to pursue our personal goals. Sometimes it may seem that health care professionals have blood glucose management as their only goal . . . while we are interested in the day-to-day enjoyment of life.

Ultimately, we do have the same goal, which is why we need to communicate our needs, values, and other goals to our health care providers, so they can help us fit diabetes into our lives. I like my diabetes team. They consider me the captain of the team. They are there to help me achieve the objectives I have for my life.

It is not just in some of us; it is in everyone. And as we let our light shine, we unconsciously give other people permission to do the same. As we are liberated from our own fear, our presence automatically liberates others.

—Marianne Williamson

Having a supportive health care team is absolutely essential to living well with the challenge of diabetes. Because diabetes needs to be managed on a daily, and even hourly, basis, we need support available to us outside of the clinic. We need support where we live. I am inspired by the stories of people around me who are generous enough to share how they support one another.

A retired teacher friend of ours is just such a generous and loving person. He told of the experience he and his wife had when she was being treated for cancer, and gave us insight into the remarkable human capacity to cope. Commenting on her baldness following chemotherapy, he said, "There's more of her to kiss."

The essential element of the uniquely human way of life was the economic pact between suppliers of meat and suppliers of vegetables . . . .Sharing, not hunting or gathering as such, is what made us human.

—Richard Leakey

My friend and mentor, Reverend Robert Esbjornson, is well-acquainted with diabetes. His daughter has had it for more than 40 years, his son has had it for 20 years, and his wife had it for many years prior to her death from breast cancer.

His perspective includes not only that of a person standing by, but also a professional with more than 30 years experience as a professor of medical ethics. He has thought deeply about life with diabetes. One conclusion he has reached is that the basic strategy for care is not that of a warrior making war on an ailment. Rather, we are the diplomat engaged in ongoing negotiations, accepting the condition as a fact that won't go away but that can be managed.

Diplomacy, not war. Negotiating with finesse, not fighting.

What role do you play in managing diabetes? Warrior? Diplomat? Other?

Birth and death are present in every moment.
— Thich Nhat Hanh

At the end of the play *Cyrano de Bergerac*, an old, frail Cyrano is seated beneath a tree while leaves gracefully fall down around him. The falling leaves give beauty, gentleness, and a naturalness to Cyrano's impending death. Leaves let go and fall without regret. This seasonal metaphor helps us to realize that death is not final. New life emerges from the old in another season.

Plays, poetry, music . . . the arts . . . are gifts of the spirit. Their messages lodge in our hearts and surface at times later in life when we need their instruction, insight, inspiration, and healing.

Every moment Nature starts on the longest
journey, and every moment she reaches her goal.
—Goethe

Each day we race toward Life's "finish line." It is well to pause and make note of where we are. Although you may not see this point in your journey as your version of the finish line, where you are is its own endpoint. It is a place of beauty, a place with lessons to share, joy to give, and growth to experience.

Traditional Chinese medicine promotes living in the moment, being "present" in the moment. This philosophy is greatly enhanced by the fact that the Chinese language has no past or future tense. Everything is present.

Carry that thought with you today. Each moment is its own destination.

The battles that count aren't the ones for gold medals. The struggles within yourself—the invisible, inevitable battles inside all of us— that's where it's at.

—Jesse Owens

Diabetes is largely an invisible disease. People cannot tell by looking at us that we have diabetes. The term *invisible chronicity* applies to diabetes and any other chronic condition that cannot be seen. Because our diabetes is not apparent to the people around us, the challenges we encounter in managing it are taken on within ourselves.

I have always felt a tremendous admiration for people who have diabetes. Few people understand what it means, what we do, what we face.

I think we all deserve gold medals.

*Let everyone sweep in front of her own door and
the whole world will be clean.*

—Goethe

At times the health care picture is painted as
so grim that we feel helpless to change it. But, as individuals, we can positively impact our own health, that
of our families, and that of our country. Our day-to-
day choices make a difference in our own lives, and
when we multiply healthy choices by many individuals, the impact is great.

A woman aboard an airplane had a seizure
because of low blood sugar. She was taken off the
plane by paramedics, by ambulance to a hospital, and
kept overnight. She had taken her diabetes medication that morning but didn't eat enough food. A
totally preventable problem cost the "system" thousands of dollars. A man in a restaurant took his insulin
after being told that his wait would be about 30 minutes. An hour and a half later, he awakened with a
paramedic bending over him.

Today, diabetes is one of the most expensive diseases in our nation. Preventable problems are just
that—preventable. Let each of us commit to taking
charge of our lives, taking responsibility for our
choices. We can help save the system, and we can
improve our health and future well-being.

Humor is the great thing, the saving thing.
The minute it crops up, all our irritations and
resentments slip away and a sunny spirit takes
their place.

—Mark Twain

One of Twain's endearing qualities was humor. But he also had a message to deliver, and his messages endure because they were delivered with humor. In an essay entitled *The Virtue of Vice*, he recommended that people retain a vice or two in life. He likened it to a ship's having extra cargo that it can dump over the side if a bad storm necessitated a lighter load.

Humor enables us to make a point without it sounding like a lesson.

The second half of a man's life is made up of nothing but the habits he has acquired during the first half.

—Fyodor Dostoyevsky

For those of us who have already completed the first half of our lives, this is an interesting thought to consider. What are those habits we acquired? As you reflect on them, select the ones you'd like to change or modify. What can you choose to do that is different? Are you ready to do it now?

And, for those of you who are still in the first half of your lives, what are the behavioral and mental habits you are developing? Will you be satisfied to take them with you into the second half of your life? If not, now is the time to change or modify them.

God turns you from one feeling to another and teaches by means of opposites, so that you will have two wings to fly, not one.

—Rumi

Disease and difficulty can be blessings. Without struggle, we remain weak. A great illustration of this is seen in a story of a man who raised butterflies as a hobby. He was so touched by the difficulties they had in emerging from the cocoon that, out of mistaken kindness, he once split the cocoon with his thumbnail so that the tiny creature could escape without a struggle.

That butterfly was never able to use its wings.

There are two ways of spreading light: to be the candle, or the mirror that reflects it.
—Edith Wharton

Even with an active faith, we are not towers of strength, acceptance, and peace all the time. There are times of questioning, vulnerability, anger, and sadness over disease and disability. And there are simply days when we're down. These are the times to turn to external sources of power and reignite our spirits by receiving their "spark."

Nature is a magnificent spark! Have you ever looked closely at a tree and been inspired by it? The Norway pine is one of my favorites—tall, straight, strong, and yet able to bend and sway with the wind. What a lesson can be learned from this beautiful, resilient tree!

Allow yourself to be rejuvenated through the power of nature. Open yourself to its healing effects. The cleansing fragrance of an evening rain or the beauty of the rainbow that follows can inspire a quiet peace within you. Discover that part of nature that touches you with its power.

*No athlete ever lived, or saint or poet for that
matter, who was content with what he did
yesterday, or would even bother thinking about it.
Their pure concern is the present. Why should we
common folk be different?*

—George A. Sheehan, MD

Art is surely a wonderful spark to inspire and ignite the spirit. Stories of the great artists are yet another source of inspiration. Pierre Auguste Renoir had crippling arthritis, yet he continued to paint. Henri Matisse visited the old master one day and remarked, "How can you continue to paint when you are in such great pain?"

Renoir replied simply, "The beauty remains. The pain passes."

A reporter asked Pablo Casals, the great musician, why he still practiced the cello 6 hours a day at the age of 90. "Because," said Casals, "I'm beginning to see some improvement."

*Someday after mastering the winds, the tides, and
    gravity
We shall harness for God the energy of Love
And then for the second time in history,
We shall have discovered Fire.*

—Pierre Teilhard de Chardin

Harold S. Kushner, author of *When Bad Things
Happen to Good People,* commented that the most
important ingredient in finding fulfillment is to know
that we have made a difference. He said it needn't be
something great. "Little deeds of loving kindness
make the difference." Rabbi Kushner suggested that
just as our bodies require certain kinds of food for good
health, "our souls are made so certain kinds of behaviors are healthy for us and other kinds are toxic."

Theologian Paul Tillich demonstrated the
importance of kindness when he said that God is not
a benevolent, but distant, cloud in the sky, separate
from us "down here." Instead, God is as close as the
closest human being is to us. God is in each of us, and
we connect with God whenever we communicate a
loving message to anyone around us.

The greatest revolution of our generation is the discovery that human beings, by changing the inner attitudes of their minds, can change the outer aspects of their lives.

—William James

Self-image is a powerful force in our lives. Who you *think* you are determines what you do and how you feel about yourself. A positive self-image serves a function similar to that of a coach. When your parents are no longer doing the coaching and encouraging, you can look to your own internal coach for approval and advice.

You control your self-image. No matter what negative messages you receive, you can choose the messages to accept and the ones to reject. You can change the impact of negative messages by using one of the most effective mental tools known: positive self-talk. You change the way you feel about yourself by changing your thoughts and what you say to yourself. Always say "You can do it."

He who has done his best for his own time has lived for all times.

—Johann von Schiller

The energy, devotion, and commitment that we put into our efforts to live well connect us to all those heroes who have ever lived, who did the best they could with their challenges. A child with cerebral palsy who falls on the sidewalk, then picks up his crutches, stands and continues his walk is as brave as any ship's captain who ever sailed through the most ferocious storm. Maybe braver.

Let me win, but if I cannot win, let me be brave in the attempt.

—Special Olympics Motto

The secret of getting ahead is getting started. The secret of getting started is breaking your complex overwhelming tasks into small, manageable tasks, and then starting on the first one.

—Mark Twain

Here is another example of how the wisdom that gives direction to life can be focused on diabetes. It's natural for people to feel overwhelmed when facing a new challenge: going from pills to insulin, starting a new meal plan, or embarking on an exercise program. But by breaking the challenge into manageable tasks, it is less daunting. With an exercise program, for instance, getting started may be as simple as walking to the end of the block and back. Then you can start to build up your distance or time and speed until you can walk briskly for 30 minutes a day, five days a week. It may take you a year to get to that goal, but that year will pass anyway . . . won't you be glad to have something new to show for it?

No one can persuade another to change. Each of us guards a gate of change that can only be opened from the inside.

—Marilyn Ferguson

Well-meaning health care professionals often try to persuade their patients to make lifestyle changes. But change will occur only if an individual makes that choice for himself or herself. Are there changes that you would like to make in your eating and exercise habits? Are there changes you would like to see in yourself (perhaps in your weight, energy level, blood sugar control, or cholesterol levels)? What can you do to make the change occur?

Remember the 10 most powerful two-letter words: If it is to be, it is up to me.

Mix a little foolishness with your prudence: it's good to be silly at the right moment.

—Horace

Take a pad of self-stick notes and write messages that are both humorous and meaningful, like: "Exercise and Diet to Fight Hazardous Waists!" Other reminders include "Breathe," since deep breathing is important in lowering blood pressure and stress management, or "Smile" because the body releases endorphins (a natural pain killer and mood enhancer) when we smile.

Put these notes where you can see them every day.

Ultimately, the only power to which man should
aspire is that which he exercises over himself.
—Elie Wiesel

Diabetes is described as the most "patient-managed" disease because the person who has it is responsible for controlling it on a day-to-day and an hour-by-hour basis. We can blame external factors—from poor food selections in the employee cafeteria to bad weather that cancels our outdoor walk—for making it difficult for us to manage our diabetes well. But although we cannot control these external factors, we *can* control ourselves. We can bring lunch to work and walk in an indoor shopping mall or a heated, underground garage. We can choose thoughts that will inspire us to take charge of life.

And the day came when the risk it took to remain tight in the bud was more painful than the risk it took to blossom.

—Anais Nin

The risks of staying where we are can include:

- remaining on one or two shots of insulin when "blossoming" (to prevent a rising A1C) would require three or four or an insulin pump
- continuing to check your urine for glucose readings instead of using a blood glucose meter
- staying on the same ineffective oral hypo-glycemic agent instead of trying the new ones
- following old eating habits instead of updating your food plan

Blossoming can mean opening yourself to a long list of activities from your pre-diagnosis days, such as resuming travel and social activities, or it can mean finding new pleasures, such as sports.

Ask yourself: Are you still tight in the bud? Is the old way of doing things no longer working for you? Is it keeping you from feeling better?

Listening is a magnetic and strange thing, a creative force. The friends who listen to us are the ones we move toward, and we want to sit in their radius. When we are listened to, it creates us, makes us unfold and expand.

—Karl Menninger

Our lives are stories. We are storytellers who need listeners in order to continue the development of our stories, and thus, our lives. The simple act of telling our stories provides us with heightened self-awareness. We can know what we think and how we feel. With this awareness, we can make decisions about the direction to take next.

We are our choices

—Jean-Paul Sartre

Beyond the obvious behavioral choices of what we eat, whether we exercise or not, and how we cope with stress, what are the choices we have made (and continue to make) that define us? Be sure to include your favorite personal philosophies in response to that question.

If you share this insight with a friend or group of friends, you will be telling your story and learning even more about the choices you have made, why you made them, and how they have shaped you.

Laughter is to life what shock absorbers are to automobiles. It won't take the potholes out of the road, but it sure makes the ride smoother.
—Barbara Johnson

Barbara's book *Humor Me* is an excellent source of laugh-provoking insights. One of my favorites is: "If it's true that we are what we eat, then I am fast, easy, and cheap!"

Laughter gives us distance. It allows us to step back from an event, deal with it, and then move on.
—Bob Newhart

Sometimes we see the absurdity of an event right away, and we can't help but laugh. But other times we need to get some distance between ourselves and the stresses that surround us. Laughter can help to give us that distance and can serve as a shock absorber. I have always felt that if I can laugh, then I am stronger than whatever is stressing me.

When at last I took the time to look into the heart of a flower, it opened up a whole new world—a world where every country walk would be an adventure, where every garden would become an enchanted one.

—Princess Grace of Monaco

What activities in your life help transport you from the mundane to the marvelous? Looking into the heart of a flower may not work for you. Perhaps what works for you is watching a professional athlete—whether it's a football player or a golfer or a gymnast—move with precision and grace.

Diabetes management doesn't have to be the focus of your days. The focus of each day is the wonder, joy, and fulfillment that can be found when we really seek meaning in our moments. *Life* is the focus of our lives. Diabetes management is really just a task we need to complete so that we can enjoy life.

Progress always involves risks. You can't steal second base and keep your foot on first.
—Frederick B. Wilcox

One of the measurements of progress in diabetes is the new treatments and guidelines, such as the recommendations for nutrition and exercise. Many of us resist anything new because we've gotten comfortable with the way we've always done things. What are the risks involved if you change the way you've always done something? List them. What are the potential rewards you could experience? List them. Using the Ben Franklin system of weighing risks and benefits, which action makes more sense?

Let us go singing as far as we go; the road will be less tedious.

—Virgil

If we view the road as a metaphor for our lives, the "singing" can be anything we focus on to add pleasure to our daily journey through life. It can be people (friends new and old), events (whether we participate or observe), or activities (even singing!). The tedium of daily blood sugar monitoring can be seen in a different light when it's done to enable us to participate in an activity we enjoy.

Opportunity is missed by most people because it is dressed in overalls, and looks like work.
—Thomas A. Edison

When I first heard about blood glucose monitoring, all I could think of was the finger-stick blood tests and how much they hurt! For me, this opportunity to gain real control over my life and to be able to participate more fully in life looked like only pain.

Fortunately, I met with a diabetes nurse educator who taught me the proper technique (which was much less painful) and helped me realize the far-reaching power of blood glucose monitoring. Using the information I get from monitoring, I can manage my diabetes and no longer have to allow diabetes to manage my life. And now that we know that well-managed diabetes can prevent the drastic complications of diabetes, the dark veil that once hung over my future has been lifted.

All the darkness of the world cannot put out the light of one small candle.

—Anonymous

*H*ope is the light of that one small candle. What does your hope hinge upon? Does your hope rest on technology, like blood glucose monitoring, new medications or delivery systems, and research on islet cell transplantation, or on the knowledge that you have the best in medical care? Does your hope go beyond the tangible to include a strong faith that tells you, convincingly and unequivocally, that no matter what the future holds, you will do well?

I get wisdom day and night
Turning darkness into light.

from *The Scholar and His Cat*
translator, Robin Flower

A well-spent day brings happy sleep.
—Leonardo da Vinci

Wisdom is a thread that connects us to one another, whether we are contemporaries sharing similar experiences or people of different cultures and eras sharing ideas. Leonardo's observation could easily be our own. We each have our own definition of a well-spent day, one that is unique to each of us. What is included in your definition or description of a "well-spent day"? How is today measuring up so far?

To engage with honor the full possibility of your life is to engage in a worthy way the possibility of your new day. Each day is different.
—John O'Donohue

Ill habits gather by unseen degrees,
As brooks make rivers, rivers run to seas.
—John Dryden

Not only do bad habits just sort of creep up on us, but our good habits depart by the same unseen manner. Take a moment to review your lifestyle and behavior. Are you eating nutritiously most of the time? How are you doing in restaurants? What items do you routinely put in your grocery cart? What about your activity level? Are you cutting back on activity because your life has gotten increasingly busy? Would you describe your lifestyle as healthy? If not, are there a few changes you want to make? What is stopping you?

What we hope ever to do with ease, we must learn to do with diligence.

—Samuel Johnson

Once you have chosen a behavior that you would like to become a habit, make a goal that you can measure. An example is "I will walk 30 minutes a day Monday, Tuesday, Wednesday, Thursday, and Saturday." Then, to remind you, put a small, colored dot (you can get them at office supply stores or drugstores) in strategic locations where you will see them frequently. Places to put dot reminders include: the TV remote control (bright orange there!), bathroom mirror, computer screen, refrigerator door (red dot there?), your watch, your calendar or daily planner, your checkbook, and your car's steering wheel or dashboard.

Think of small, fun rewards to give yourself for each week that you accumulate 150 minutes of walking. Maybe start a "150 Minute" club at work. The Diabetes Prevention Program (DPP) showed that a 7% weight loss and 150 minutes per week of exercise prevented the development of diabetes in people at risk. For those who already have diabetes, 150 minutes of walking helps you manage blood sugar levels and your weight, and keep your heart healthy. Let's lace up those shoes!

I count him braver who conquers his desires than him who conquers his enemies; for the hardest victory is the victory over self.

—Aristotle

Without hesitation or embarrassment, list some of the victories, even small ones, you have had over yourself. To get you started, consider some of these:

- resisting tempting food
- going on a walk when you'd prefer to stay in bed
- saying "no" to second helpings of food that tasted really good
- refusing to allow negative thoughts to rule you
- choosing healthy strategies like laughter or exercise to manage stress
- coming to peace with the fact that you have diabetes—with no more denial

What experiences can you add?

I know the price of success: dedication, hard work, and an unremitting devotion to the things you want to happen.

—Frank Lloyd Wright

Whether it's building a magnificent house or building a healthy life, the price is the same.

He who distinguishes the true savor of his food can never be a glutton; he who does not, cannot be otherwise.

—Henry David Thoreau

We eat so fast! Slow down. Put your fork down between bites. *Savor the taste.* Just for today, try to take your time and enjoy it. Then ask yourself, "What if 'just for today' became a habit, something I did every-day?" Try it! See what happens.

A strong positive mental attitude will create more miracles than any wonder drug.

—Patricia Neal

Actress Patricia Neal had a severe, debilitating stroke from which she recovered. She credits a positive attitude with creating this miracle. Centuries earlier, the French dramatist Moliere commented: "The mind has great influence over the body, and maladies often have their origin there." What evidence have you seen or experienced that has shaped your opinion on the power of the mind?

*When I hear music I fear no danger; I am
invulnerable, I see no foe.*
—Henry David Thoreau

What role does music play in your life? What
types of music do you enjoy when you want to relax?
Do you use music to augment a mood? To change it?
Is music one of the ways you manage stress?

The highest reward for a person's toil is not what they get for it, but what they become by it.
—John Ruskin

In another era, another culture, we hear a similar philosophy expressed a little differently.

Honey, if it don't kill ya, it'll make ya a better person.
—Lou's Grandma
Dr. Lou Bellamy is a professor of theater
at the University of Minnesota

If you hear a voice within you saying, 'You are not a painter," then by all means paint . . . and that voice will be silenced.

—Vincent Van Gogh

Sometimes those voices come at us from the outside. Sometimes they say that diabetes is a reason why we cannot do a certain thing or become something. Those voices can be silenced as well. Do it. Be it.

A book is like a garden carried in a pocket.
—Chinese proverb

When you need a reward for a positive change you have made, or when you have saved up a few dollars, visit your favorite bookstore and find the section where they have pocket-sized books. Buy several and carry one with you at all times. Waiting need never be a chore when you have your own garden to enjoy . . . right in your pocket.

Health is the first muse, and sleep is the condition to produce it.

—Ralph Waldo Emerson

If today were your 100th birthday and someone were to ask you how you've lived so long, what are the "conditions" you would include in your answer? You may want to express this as a little story. "From the time I was a small child I always . . . and I never . . . Then, as I grew into adulthood I began to . . .

Happy Birthday. Wishing you many happy, healthy returns!

I believe that we are solely responsible for our choices.

—Elisabeth Kubler-Ross

I believe our choices depend on a foundation of knowledge and skills about how to manage our diabetes and on an equally good base of knowledge and skills about how to manage ourselves. Self-management goes hand in hand with mental and spiritual well-being and enables us to clarify our values, set goals, solve problems, cope with the stresses of life, get support, and stay motivated.

In the book of life, the answers aren't in the back.
　　　　　　—Charlie Brown (Charles Schulz)

Life's most profound questions do not have answers. Asking questions can bring insights, but no answers. Becoming philosophical about life is the approach used in the book *Plato, not Prozac! Applying Eternal Wisdom to Everyday Problems* by Lou Martinoff. Martinoff says that "by getting a handle on their personal philosophies of life, sometimes with the help of the great thinkers of the past, people can build a framework for managing whatever they face and go into the next situation more solidly grounded and spiritually or philosophically whole."

This is what we come here to do.

To be a philosopher is not merely to have subtle thoughts, nor even to found a school . . . . It is to solve some of the problems of life, not theoretically, but practically.

—Henry David Thoreau

Throughout this book are ideas from ancient and contemporary philosophers. These thoughts are here to stimulate your thinking and lead you to useful insights. They may also lead you to practical solutions and action. Another philosopher says:

The way I see it, if you want the rainbow, you gotta put up with the rain.

—Dolly Parton

Dolly Parton has established Imagination Library, an educational foundation to provide free books to children. She has now given away one million books.

Now what's your philosophy in the metaphoric rain that you are currently facing? What is your rainbow, the one that inspires you to keep slogging through the rain?

Success is 99 percent failure.
—Soichiro Honda, Founder,
Honda Motor Corp.

Each failure has a lesson to teach. We learn what didn't work. The results of blood glucose monitoring are not indicators that *you* have succeeded or failed. They give you an important message about the success or failure of *your regimen*. Blood glucose results give you information you can use to make choices and feel better.

The world is all gates, all opportunities, strings of tension waiting to be struck.
—Ralph Waldo Emerson

Has diabetes changed your worldview? Do you see fewer opportunities ahead because you have diabetes? If so, think again. Gary Hall Jr., who has type 1 diabetes, won several Olympic gold medals after being diagnosed with the disease. Halle Berry won an Academy Award after her diagnosis. Throughout the world, in our everyday lives, there are unrecognized heroes with diabetes who follow their dreams and, striking tense strings, produce beautiful music.

Let your hook be always cast. In the stream where you least expect it, there will be fish.

—Ovid

You would not expect to find much good in a disease like diabetes. If it were a stream, would it be an unending torrent of deprivation, needles, and complications? Or could you see diabetes as that metaphoric stream that yields friendships, careers, meaningful volunteer experiences, and powerful personal growth? Cast your hook. Cast again. Keep dreaming and believing.

Gray skies are just clouds passing over.
—Duke Ellington

During long periods of gray weather, people can experience a type of depression known as SAD, or seasonal affective disorder. Have you ever experienced it? Does it help you to think of it as a temporary condition, like clouds passing over? Awareness of the disorder can help you cope with this mood-altering experience. Awareness of what's causing you to feel down can lead you to remedies, such as adding more light to your rooms, getting together with friends who add light to your life, and seeking resources such as funny movies and cheerful music to call forth the light within you. Activities such as these can restore your hope.

In the land of hope, there is never any winter.
—Russian proverb

When my subject is being effective, I am glad, and when it is worriedly procrastinating, I am sad. When it makes mistakes, I learn the most and am elated. That is the extent of my prejudice.
　　　　—Buckminster Fuller on observing himself

The study of ourselves is the quest and the task for which we were born. Learning who we are and then learning to enjoy who we are is a full time job. Do enjoy it.

There is a vitality, a life force, an energy, a quickening, that is translated through you into action, and because there is only one of you in all time, this expression is unique.
　　　　—Martha Graham

In times of profound change, the learners inherit the earth, while the learned find themselves beautifully equipped to deal with a world that no longer exists.
—Al Rogers

I learned about courage, faith, and determination from my mother. The day after Dad's funeral, she invited my 12-year-old brother and me to join her as she drove the car around the block. She had never driven a car before. Her message was clear: Life goes on. Each of us has things to learn and things to do while we are here that no one else can do for us.

In the past 10 years, we have learned so much about managing diabetes. If you haven't been to a diabetes class in years, or ever, now is the time to go. There is much that is wonderful and powerful for you to learn and to use.

Music washes away the dust of everyday life from your feet.

—Wynton Marsalis

A woman stranded alone at night on a mountain in freezing temperatures and falling snow on Christmas Eve knew it was dance or die. So, she danced in the dark, playing tunes in her head, until dawn Christmas Day, when rescuers found her.

She danced to keep warm, to stay awake . . . to live.

What a wonderfully heroic story! As I read it in the newspaper, I thought of the times over the years when I have been stranded in various places . . . usually airports. I thought about how grateful I was to have my blood glucose meter, insulin, and extra food. I've always made it through these experiences . . . sometimes with a begrudging spirit. This story helped me to see that I can do more than merely "make it." I can survive with joy . . . with body, mind, and soul intact.

Along with granola bars, I shall add music to my survival kit.

My kitchen is a mystical place, a kind of temple for me. It is a place where the surfaces seem to have significance, where the sounds and odors carry meaning that transfers from the past and bridges to the future.

—Pearl Bailey

Laugher is brightest where food is best.

—Irish proverb

Perhaps the greatest gift of our winter celebration is the coming together of family and friends to share food, talk, music, and laughter. Once more we have an opportunity to give each other our attention and our respect. We can also give our attention and respect to the food we prepare, the stories we tell each other, and the songs we sing. I think that these may last longer than the presents we might buy and exchange.

If you have no family or friends nearby, there are soup kitchens that need your helping hands or donation from your kitchen; there are family shelters where children appreciate good food or having a book read to them. There are people in nursing homes and hospitals who would enjoy a gift from your kitchen or your visit. If you want to give, you will find a way. You can start with giving a smile to each person you meet.

Come, Whoever you are! Wanderer, worshipper,
lover of leaving
Come. This is not a caravan of despair. It doesn't
matter if you've broken your vow a thousand
times, still
Come, and yet again, come.

—Rumi

Consider the wisdom in the *Creed for Optimists* by Christian D. Larsen:

- Talk health, happiness, and prosperity to every person you meet.
- Make all your friends feel there is something special in them.
- Be as enthusiastic about the success of others as you are about your own.
- Forgive the mistakes of the past.

Be kind, for everyone you meet is fighting a hard battle.

—Plato

We all wear masks. Sometimes we hide behind them because we don't want others to know that we are hurting or afraid or lacking in self-confidence. Or, sometimes we put on a mask to help us play any of the roles we have in life. (If we look the part, we'll be successful in the role?)

Behind every mask however, is a person, who at any given moment, may be struggling. If the Golden Rule still holds true, Plato's advice should, too.

A human being should be able to change a diaper, plan an invasion, butcher a hog, conn a ship, design a building, write a sonnet, balance accounts, build a wall, set a bone, comfort the dying, take orders, give orders, cooperate, act alone, pitch manure, solve equations, analyze a new problem, program a computer, cook a tasty meal, fight efficiently, die gallantly. Specialization is for insects.

—Robert A. Heinlein

Never stop learning and growing. Check to be sure that you are living your life fully. Go learn to do new things, and count your wealth in experiences. These are the only things besides your body that you truly own.

The repetition in nature may not be a mere recurrence.
It may be a theatrical "encore."

—G. K. Chesterton

I like the idea that it is my "Encore!" that brings the seasons of the spirit back on the stage again and again. My choice has brought about their return. Courage, Faith, Wisdom, and Joy do not automatically recur in my life. I choose to invite their powerful, yet peace-giving, presence. The words "theatrical encore" tell me that this is not a whisper. We shout ENCORE! There is neither timidity nor confusion. My desire for these spiritual values is utterly clear.

Wisdom guides my choice each time I shout ENCORE for Courage, Faith, and Joy. And Joy. I need Joy. I want Joy. ENCORE!

Laughter is the sun that drives winter from the human face.

—Victor Hugo

Ancient wisdom and modern research supports the idea that laughter is good medicine. Legendary comedian Milton Berle said, "Laughter is an instant vacation." That wisdom is made real in the life of a friend of mine who rents funny movies when he is feeling down and wants to get back up.

I think of what a gift this friend is to me because he loves to laugh, and he laughs a lot. When he laughs, he lifts all of us who are with him. We can see the sun in his face and feel its warmth in our hearts. I cherish my friends who make me laugh. Thanks, Mike.

P.S. Winter with such short days and long nights is a good season for seeing funny movies or reading funny books. I laughed so hard when I read the essay on the mother of the bride in a Robert Fulghum book that I cried . . . which was a little embarrassing because I was sitting alone on an airplane.

Why does anybody tell a story? It does indeed have something to do with faith, faith that the universe has meaning, that our little human lives are not irrelevant, that what we choose to say or do matters, matters cosmically.

—Madeleine L'Engle

According to Dr. Remen, author of *Kitchen Table Wisdom,* "Everyone is a story." Over the past 30 years, I have shared my thoughts and stories with thousands of people here and abroad. The reward I cherish is that people share their stories with me. I believe what Joseph Campbell said, "We shall come to the center of our own existence and, where we had thought to be alone, we shall be with all the world."

When you are aware of your own story, you can realize the power you have because you are the author of the story.

I continue talking with God. Each day, many times each day, I ask for guidance or I offer thanks. And I listen. As a seeker of meaning, I have come to understand that there are no final answers. We are given insights into how we can cope with challenges, how we can weave difficulty and joy into the tapestry of our lives. Our worldview expands as we develop a philosophy that allows this, and our stories are so much richer.

Blessings on you and your story.

About the American Diabetes Association

The American Diabetes Association is the nation's leading voluntary health organization supporting diabetes research, information, and advocacy. Its mission is to prevent and cure diabetes and to improve the lives of all people affected by diabetes. The American Diabetes Association is the leading publisher of comprehensive diabetes information. Its huge library of practical and authoritative books for people with diabetes covers every aspect of self-care—cooking and nutrition, fitness, weight control, medications, complications, emotional issues, and general self-care.

To order American Diabetes Association books: Call 1-800-232-6733. Or log on to http://store.diabetes.org

To join the American Diabetes Association: Call 1-800-806-7801. www.diabetes.org/membership

For more information about diabetes or ADA programs and services: Call 1-800-342-2383. E-mail: AskADA@diabetes.org or log on to www.diabetes.org

To locate an ADA/NCQA Recognized Provider of quality diabetes care in your area: www.ncqa.org/dprp/

To find an ADA Recognized Education Program in your area: Call 1-888-232-0822. www.diabetes.org/recognition/education.asp

To join the fight to increase funding for diabetes research, end discrimination, and improve insurance coverage: Call 1-800-342-2383. www.diabetes.org/advocacy

To find out how you can get involved with the programs in your community: Call 1-800-342-2383. See below for program Web addresses.

- *American Diabetes Month:* Educational activities aimed at those diagnosed with diabetes—month of November. www.diabetes.org/ADM
- *American Diabetes Alert:* Annual public awareness campaign to find the undiagnosed—held the fourth Tuesday in March. www.diabetes.org/alert
- *The Diabetes Assistance & Resources Program (DAR):* diabetes awareness program targeted to the Latino community. www.diabetes.org/DAR
- *African American Program:* diabetes awareness program targeted to the African American community. www.diabetes.org/africanamerican
- *Awakening the Spirit: Pathways to Diabetes Prevention & Control:* diabetes awareness program targeted to the Native American community. www.diabetes.org/awakening

To find out about an important research project regarding type 2 diabetes: www.diabetes.org/ada/research.asp

To obtain information on making a planned gift or charitable bequest: Call 1-888-700-7029. www.diabetes.org/ada/plan.asp
To make a donation or memorial contribution: Call 1-800-342-2383. www.diabetes.org/ada/cont.asp